**Essentials
of Vascular
Laboratory
Diagnosis**

To my immediate and extended family for their continued support and encouragement, to my mentors for their advice and guidance, and to the vascular sonographers at the University of Pennsylvania Health System for their compassionate care and team effort. *Emile R. Mohler III.*

To my husband and daughter, Mark and Mia, for their ongoing support and encouragement, and to all the vascular sonographers at Brigham and Women's Hospital who continue to inspire me. *Marie Gerhard-Hermann.*

To my incredible wife and outstanding daughters, whose patience is only matched by their love for their crazy husband and father. *Michael Jaff.*

Essentials of Vascular Laboratory Diagnosis

EDITED BY

Emile R. Mohler III, MD

Director, Vascular Medicine
University of Pennsylvania School of Medicine
Philadelphia

Marie Gerhard-Herman, MD

Medical Director, Vascular Diagnostic Laboratory
Brigham and Women's Hospital, Harvard Medical School,
Boston, Massachusetts

Michael R. Jaff, DO

Medical Director, Vascular Ultrasound Core Laboratory
Massachusetts General Hospital,
Boston, Massachusetts

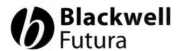

© 2005 by Blackwell Publishing
Blackwell Futura is an imprint of Blackwell Publishing

Blackwell Publishing, Inc., 350 Main Street, Malden, Massachusetts 02148-5020, USA
Blackwell Publishing Ltd, 9600 Garsington Road, Oxford OX4 2DQ, UK
Blackwell Science Asia Pty Ltd, 550 Swanston Street, Carlton, Victoria 3053, Australia

First published 2005

ISBN-13: 978-1-4051-2215-3
ISBN-10: 1-4051-2215-3

Library of Congress Cataloging-in-Publication Data

Essentials of vascular laboratory diagnosis / edited by Emile R. Mohler
III, Marie Gerhard-Herman, Michael R. Jaff.
    p. ; cm.
  Includes bibliographical references and index.
  ISBN-13: 978-1-4051-0382-4 (alk. paper)
  ISBN-10: 1-4051-0382-5 (alk. paper)
  1. Blood-vessels—Diseases—Diagnosis. 2. Diagnosis, Laboratory.
3. Blood-vessels—Ultrasonic imaging.
  [DNLM: 1. Vascular Diseases—diagnosis. 2. Diagnostic Techniques,
Cardiovascular. 3. Ultrasonography, Doppler—methods.] I. Mohler, Emile R.
II. Gerhard-Herman, Marie.
III. Jaff, Michael R.

  RC691.5.E85 2005
  616.1'3075—dc22

2004029972

A catalogue record for this title is available from the British Library

Acquisitions: Gina Almond
Development Editor: Karen Moore

Set in 9.5/12 Palatino by SNP Best-set Typesetter Ltd, Hong Kong
Printed and bound in India by Replika Press Pvt. Ltd, Kundli

For further information on Blackwell Publishing, visit our website:
www.blackwellcardiology.com

Notice: The indications and dosages of all drugs in this book have been recommended
in the medical literature and conform to the practices of the general community. The
medications described do not necessarily have specific approval by the Food and Drug
Administration for use in the diseases and dosages for which they are recommended.
The package insert for each drug should be consulted for use and dosage as approved
by the FDA. Because standards for usage change, it is advisable to keep abreast of
revised recommendations, particularly those concerning new drugs.

Contents

List of Contributors

Ferdinando S. Buonanno, MD
Assistant Professor, Stroke Service, Massachusetts General Hospital and Harvard Medical School, Boston, Massachusetts

Jeffrey P. Carpenter, MD
Professor of Surgery, University of Pennsylvania School of Medicine; and Director, Vascular Laboratory, Hospital of the University of Pennsylvania, Philadelphia

Julia T. Davis, MS, RN, RVT
Technical Director, Vascular Laboratory, Hospital of the University of Pennsylvania, Philadelphia

Karen Lisa Furie, MD, MPH
Associate Professor, Stroke Service, Massachusetts General Hospital and Harvard Medical School, Boston, Massachusetts

Marie Gerhard-Herman, MD
Medical Director, Vascular Diagnostic Laboratory, Brigham and Women's Hospital, Harvard Medical School, Boston, Massachusetts

John Gocke, MD, MPH, RVT
Medical Director, Vascular Laboratory, Midwest Heart Specialists; and Medical Director, Vascular Laboratory, La Grange Memorial Hospital, Downers Grove, Illinois

Corey K. Goldman, MD
Director of Vascular Medicine, Department of Cardiology, Ochsner Heart and Vascular Institute, New Orleans, Louisiana

Michael R. Jaff, DO
Medical Director, Vascular Ultrasound Core Laboratory, Massachusetts General Hospital, Boston, Massachusetts

J. Philip Kistler, MD
Professor in Neurology, Stroke Service, Massachusetts General Hospital and Harvard Medical School, Boston, Massachusetts

Itzhak Kronzon, MD
Professor of Medicine, New York University School of Medicine; and Director, Non-Invasive Cardiology, New York University Medical Center, New York

Mark E. Lockhart, MD, MPH
Assistant Professor, Department of Radiology, University of Alabama at Birmingham, Birmingham, Alabama

Thanila A. Macedo, MD
Consultant, Department of Radiology, Mayo Clinic College of Medicine, Rochester, Minnesota

Emile R. Mohler III, MD
Associate Professor of Medicine, University of Pennsylvania School of Medicine; and Director, Vascular Medicine Program, University of Pennsylvania Health System, Philadelphia

Sanjay Rajagopalan, MD
Director, Clinical Cardiovascular MRI and CT Imaging Program, Mount Sinai School of Medicine, New York

Michelle L. Robbin, MD
Professor and Chief of Ultrasound, Department of
Radiology, University of Alabama at Birmingham,
Birmingham, Alabama

Eric Edward Smith, MD
Instructor in Neurology, Stroke Service,
Massachusetts General Hospital and Harvard
Medical School, Boston, Massachusetts

Paul A. Tunick, MD
Professor of Medicine, New York University School
of Medicine, New York

Madhu B. Vijayappa, MD
Stroke Fellow, Stroke Service, Massachusetts
General Hospital and Harvard Medical School,
Boston, Massachusetts

Edward Y. Woo, MD
Assistant Professor of Surgery, Division of Vascular
Surgery, University of Pennsylvania, Philadelphia

Foreword

Although atherosclerosis is well recognized as a silent and deadly disease, cardiologists are perhaps less likely to acknowledge that it is also a systemic disease, manifesting as unique clinical syndromes when present in noncoronary circulations. Similarly, although board certified in Cardiovascular Diseases (emphasis added), many cardiologists have historically limited their practices to heart disease. Recently, driven by both a deeper understanding of vascular biology and a new found ability to perform therapeutic interventions in the peripheral vasculature, the scope of practice of cardiology has widened to encompass all of cardiovascular medicine.

However, focusing only on procedures may lead to neglect of the patient and of the critically important roles of diagnostic testing and medical treatment in caring for those with vascular disease. Individuals performing peripheral interventions or surgery must become familiar with the techniques used to detect the diseases they propose to treat, including their strengths and weaknesses, pearls and pitfalls in their performance and interpretation, and their application to patient care. In other words, cardiologists, or rather cardiovascular medicine specialists, should be just as familiar with peripheral vascular diagnostic tests as they are with echocardiography.

For cardiologists newly involved in providing care to patients with peripheral vascular disease, this text, *Essentials of Vascular Laboratory Diagnosis*, is an important contribution to their already changing scope of cardiovascular practice. This group is not small—an American Society of Echocardiography membership survey in 2003 suggested that the majority were either already performing peripheral ultrasound or anticipated doing so within 2 years. For others more familiar with the field, including radiologists, neurologists, and vascular surgeons, this book provides a welcome, comprehensive review of the topic, complete with all-important images and case presentations to better convey how this knowledge applies to patient care. It will be a valuable resource, in both the office and 'noninvasive' cardiovascular laboratory, to aid in the diagnosis and assessment of the large and growing number of patients with undiagnosed and un- or under-treated peripheral vascular disease.

Pamela S. Douglas, MD
June 2004

Preface

The diagnosis of vascular disease, primarily due to atherosclerosis and thrombosis, is based on several imaging modalities, including physiologic measurements, ultrasound imaging, x-ray-based radiographic imaging, and magnetic resonance imaging. The goal of this book is to provide a comprehensive resource for those interested in vascular diagnostic testing of the arterial and venous peripheral circulation and cerebrovascular circulation.

Traditional textbooks have been limited in their ability to provide representative images obtained during vascular testing, only providing a snapshot of clinical information. This text is directly linked to a CD which contains not only static images with clinical vignettes, but also moving images displaying the dynamic aspects of vascular pathology.

We hope that you will find the book a succinct reference tool, providing "essential" information on noninvasive methods for the diagnosis of vascular disease and proving to be a valuable reference which will be used frequently in the vascular laboratory.

We thank Boston Scientific Corporation and Cordis Endovascular, a Johnson & Johnson Company, for their support in this endeavor, allowing us to include the CD.

Principles and Instrumentation

PART 1

Principles and
Instrumentation

CHAPTER 1

1 Principles of Vascular Laboratory Testing

Marie Gerhard-Herman

Vascular laboratory testing is performed in order to examine defined blood vessels and to characterize blood flow within these vessels. This requires an understanding of vascular anatomy, ultrasound imaging, physiologic factors governing blood flow, and display of Doppler analysis.

Ultrasound image generation

An ultrasound transducer generates sound waves in discrete pulses, which then travel through the soft tissue. A fraction of the sound waves is reflected back towards the transducer as it encounters a change in tissue acoustic properties. The position of the tissue interface encountered by the returning echo is determined by the duration of time between the transmission and return of the pulse. The strength of the returning signal is proportional to the density and size of the tissue causing the scatter. The strength and time of the returning echoes are used to construct the gray scale (B mode) image. Higher transducer frequency results in greater near-field contrast resolution and decreased depth of penetration as a result of attenuation. Specular reflection occurs when an interface is large and smooth with respect to the transmitted wavelength. Specular reflection is maximal when the ultrasound beam is perpendicular to the interface, and allows for the characterization of the vessel wall.

Images of the vessel wall may also be improved by the use of harmonics. The wide bandwidth of current vascular probes allows the analysis of returning harmonics (whole number multiples) of the fundamental frequency. Conventional ultrasound imaging sends out a fundamental sound wave of defined frequency and receives the same frequency range back in the returning echoes. The fundamental wave becomes distorted as the tissue compresses and expands in response to the sound wave. This distortion results in the generation of harmonics, additional frequencies that are multiples of the emitted frequency. The receiver can detect both the original frequency and the harmonics. When the receiver detects echoes only at the harmonic frequency, it can reduce artifacts associated with the fundamental frequency, such as speckle, reverberation, and side lobes[1] (Figure 1.1).

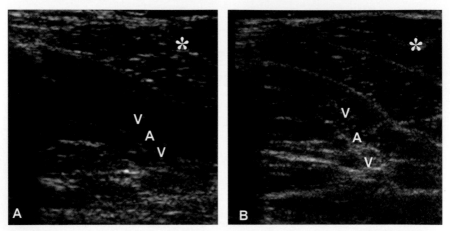

Figure 1.1 Gray scale (B mode) imaging. (A) Gray scale imaging of the posterior tibial vessels (VAV) in the calf utilizing the fundamental frequency. Near-field contrast and speckle (*) are both more evident with the fundamental frequency. (B) Imaging of the same posterior tibial vessels utilizing harmonics. The near-field resolution and speckle (*) are decreased. All interfaces appear more prominent. In this instance, harmonics allows improved detection of the posterior tibial artery and the paired posterior tibial veins.

Blood flow

Blood flow occurs when there is a difference in pressure between two points, and flow proceeds in the direction of the lower pressure[2]. Major regulation of flow occurs at the heart and at the resistance vessels. The cardiac pump cyclically restores high-pressure (high-energy) flow into the arterial system. Some energy is then lost by friction as blood flows through the arteries. The next major control point in regulating blood flow is the resistance vessels. Constriction of these vessels increases distal pressure and therefore decreases blood flow, while dilation decreases distal pressure and allows an increase in blood flow. The dynamic change possible at the level of the resistance vessels allows for a more precise regional control of blood flow to specific organs. Downstream from the resistance arterioles is the venous pool. Blood flow at this point in the system is at low pressure (energy). Venous flow is therefore more profoundly affected by the contribution of hydrostatic and intrathoracic pressures. The downstream veins are progressively larger in diameter and easily distensible; therefore, there is little resistance to forward flow. The lowest pressure (energy) in the circulatory system is in the right atrium, which normally is close to atmospheric pressure.

Laminar and nonlaminar flow

In a straight vessel with uniform diameter, blood moves forward in concentric circles with the middle circle having the highest velocity and the outermost circle having the lowest velocity. The velocity profile across the vessel is a

Laminar

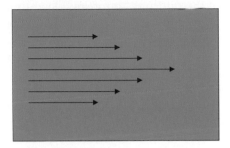

Nonlaminar

Figure 1.2 Laminar flow is characterized by the highest velocity in the center stream (long arrow) and the lowest velocity at the wall (short arrow), with a parabolic decline in velocity from mid-stream to the wall edge. Nonlaminar flow includes chaotic variations in both velocity and flow direction, as demonstrated by the arrows. It results from changes in the tube diameter.

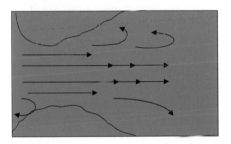

parabola, as the rate of change in velocity is greatest against the wall and least in the center. The flow velocity changes throughout the cardiac cycle, with the highest velocity during systole and the lowest velocity during diastole. There are normal and abnormal deviations from laminar flow in the circulation. The lines or circles of flow are disturbed when the vessel diameter changes and at bends or branches (Figure 1.2). Disturbances in laminar flow are referred to as turbulence[3] and are described by the dimensionless Reynolds number. Turbulence is detected on physical examination by the presence of a bruit or a thrill. Pressure decline along the length of the vessel is greater when there is turbulent flow rather than laminar flow.

Poiseuille's law

The mean velocity of laminar flow in a cylinder is directly proportional to the energy (pressure) difference between the two ends of the cylinder and to the square of the radius. The velocity is inversely proportional to the length of the tube and the blood viscosity. The most important feature of blood flow is the volume of the flow delivered, and the volume is proportional to the fourth power of the blood vessel radius. A decrease of 50% in the radius results in a 95% decrease in flow. As the length of the vessels and the viscosity of blood in the cardiovascular system do not change, it is alterations in radius and decreases in inflow pressure that limit the volume of blood flow. The resistance is the quantification of the difficulty in forcing blood through the vessels. The resistance is also derived from Poiseuille's law when the pressure differences and blood flow can be measured [4]:

Volume of flow $= [\pi(P_1 - P_2)r^4]/8L\eta$
Resistance $= 8L\eta/\pi r^4 = (P_1 - P_2)/Q$

where P is the pressure, r is the radius, L is the length, η is the viscosity, and Q is the volume flow.

Pulsatile pressure and flow

One stroke volume of blood is ejected into the arterial system with each heartbeat. The waveform of the ejected blood changes as it travels through the arterial system. During late systole, when the ejection volume decreases, the outflow volume through the peripheral resistance vessels exceeds the volume being ejected by the heart, and the pressure begins to decline. The energy stored by arterial distension also decreases throughout the cardiac cycle. The speed at which the wave travels is referred to as the pulse wave velocity. The speed of the wave is dependent on the vessel distensibility and is independent of the volume of blood flow. The amplitude of the pressure wave and the systolic pressure increase as the wave travels distally in the aorta as a result of reflected waves. Reflected waves occur with branching, changes in vessel dimensions, and changes in vascular stiffness. The reflected waves in the periphery are enhanced because of the high resistance typically encountered, and result in high thigh pressures normally greater than the ankle or brachial pressures. This is relevant to the correct interpretation of pressure measurements in peripheral arterial evaluation. As the ankle systolic pressure is normally higher than the brachial pressure, the normal ankle : brachial ratio (index) is greater than 1.0. The waveform changes when the artery is flowing into an organ with dilated resistance vessels. Forward flow is detected throughout diastole in this setting of low resistance (Figure 1.3).

Arterial stenosis

Arterial stenosis, or narrowing, can result in decreased pressure and flow downstream. A diameter decrease of 50% results in a cross-sectional area (CSA) decrease of 75%. Whether or not this results in hemodynamic change is influenced by the presence of turbulence, the ratio of stenosis CSA to more proximal CSA, the rate of flow, and the peripheral resistance. The concept of "critical stenosis" is a simplification of the complex interplay of factors. For example, serial stenoses have a greater impact on distal pressure and flow than a single stenosis. A decrease in pressure distal to the stenosis is most illustrative of the hemodynamic impact of the stenosis. Newer techniques, such as the evaluation of the

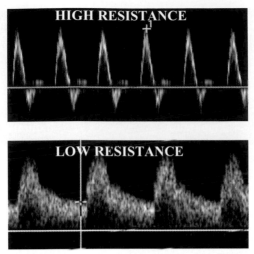

Figure 1.3 A high-resistance arterial waveform is characterized by a systolic peak and the absence of flow during some portion of diastole. A lower resistance arterial waveform is characterized by peak systolic velocity followed by continued flow during diastole until the next systolic peak.

transit of microbubbles across an organ or tissue, are also being used to determine the impact of hemodynamic alterations[5].

Venous waveforms

Phasic changes in the low-pressure venous system are a result of changes in the intrathoracic pressure with respiration and changes in right atrial pressures. The changes in flow that accompany respiration are opposite in the upper extremities when compared with the lower extremities. In the upper limbs, flow increases during inspiration, when the right atrial pressure is lowest. In the lower limbs, abdominal pressure increases during inspiration and the lower limb venous flow decreases. The amount of venous flow is also governed by the flow into the venous system. The resistance arterioles are dilated when limb blood flow increases, and venous flow therefore increases. In states of increased venous blood flow, the phasic changes may be evident (Figure 1.4). Flow and pressure changes during the cardiac cycle are most evident in the central veins[6] and are represented by three positive pressure waves. These are referred to as the a, c, and v waves and occur coincident with atrial contraction, atrial ventricular valve closure, and atrial filling, respectively. Cycle variation in the peripheral venous waveform is most evident in right heart failure when the venous pressure is increased. Cyclic variation is also apparent in healthy "well-hydrated" individuals when the venous system is fully distended.

Hydrostatic pressure and posture

Hydrostatic pressure arises from the gravitational potential energy of the blood.

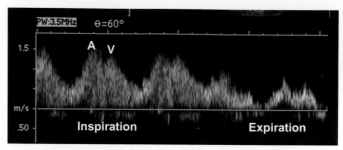

Figure 1.4 Spectral display of internal jugular venous flow. The a and v waves are evident. The velocity varies in response to the respiratory cycle, increasing during inspiration.

It occurs within the body when one part of the body is at a different elevation from another. In the upright position, the hydrostatic pressure is greatest in the lower extremities, where the additional gravitational force is the greatest. This results in venous distension and a further increase in the amount of blood pooled in the lower extremities. Contraction of the surrounding muscles increases pressure within the veins and propels blood towards the heart (as long as the one-way venous valves are competent to prevent flow away from the heart). The systolic and diastolic pressures at the ankle increase by up to 100 mmHg in the standing position, compared with the supine position, as a result of the contribution of hydrostatic pressure.

Display of Doppler information

Most images of blood flow rely on the detection and processing of Doppler shift frequencies[7]. The frequency of echoes returning after striking a moving object will be different from the frequency emitted by the transducer. The shift in frequency will be positive or negative depending on the direction of flow. The difference between the transmitted and received frequencies is affected by the speed of sound c, the flow velocity v, and the angle between the insonation beam and the direction of blood flow θ (Figure 1.5). These relationships are described by the Doppler equation:

$$f_{shift} = f_{received} - f_{transmitted} = (2f_{transmitted} \, v \cos \theta) / c$$

The Doppler angle θ therefore has a strong influence on the detected Doppler shift frequency for a given reflector velocity. In practice, the post-processing on current ultrasound machines will use the measured Doppler shift frequency to calculate the blood flow velocity:

$$v = c(f_{received} - f_{transmitted}) / 2f_{transmitted} \cos \theta$$

Spectral Doppler systems produce sound or graphic displays to represent the detected Doppler shift (Figure 1.6). The graphic displays typically have velocity

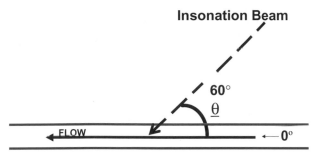

Figure 1.5 The Doppler angle refers to the angle between the insonation beam and the flow. At 0°, the insonation beam is parallel to the flow. This insonation angle is not generally achievable in vascular imaging. The angle of 60° is easily obtained in most blood vessels.

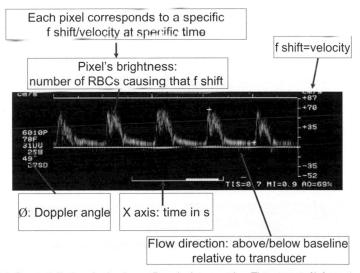

Figure 1.6 Spectral display of pulsed wave Doppler interrogation. The amount of information contained in the display is evident from a review of the many components indicated in this figure.

on the *y* axis and time on the *x* axis. Color Doppler displays the detected Doppler shift by colors indicating the velocity and direction of flow. Phasic continuous wave (CW) Doppler allows the detection of the magnitude of the Doppler shift, but not the direction. Reflectors and scatterers anywhere in the CW insonation beam contribute to the instantaneous Doppler signal. Therefore, with CW, Doppler shifts from multiple vessels can be sampled simultaneously. Pulsed wave (PW) Doppler samples and color encodes only the frequency shifts from a defined volume. The Doppler signal produced is generated from the frequency shifts (from moving targets) from one pulse echo sequence to the next. The pulse repetition frequency (PRF) must be high enough so that important details of the

Doppler signal are not lost between transmitted pulses. Aliasing occurs when Doppler shifts take place during transmitting intervals, but not during receiving intervals. The limit of the velocity display is determined by the PRF. No velocity above a specific Doppler threshold is displayed when the Doppler shift threshold is greater than one-half of the PRF. This Doppler shift threshold is referred to as the Nyquist limit. Duplex instruments allow the display of the static B mode (gray scale) image simultaneously with spectral display of the PW Doppler signal.

Doppler angle of 60°

Velocity recordings are ideally obtained with an angle of 60° between the Doppler insonation beam and the vessel wall. This is achievable and reproducible in most vascular beds (Figure 1.5). The maximal frequency shift is detected at a Doppler angle of 0°, as is used in echocardiography. This Doppler angle cannot reliably be used in vascular imaging, as the vessels are parallel rather than perpendicular to the surface. The sample volume cursor is placed parallel to the wall, and a Doppler angle from 30° to 60° between the wall and the insonation beam (or flow jet) is utilized. At angles of less than 60°, small errors in setting the angle can result in up to a 10% error in velocity estimation, while at angles of greater than 60°, small errors in setting the angle can cause up to a 25% error in the velocity estimation (Figure 1.7). The decreasing value of the cosine at the higher Doppler angles has an increasing influence on the detected Doppler shift frequency, and therefore on the velocity estimation.

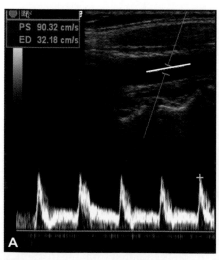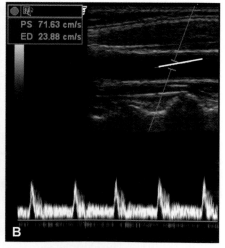

Figure 1.7 Impact of correct Doppler angle. (A) The angle between the flow and the insonation beam is 60° and the peak systolic velocity is 90.32 cm s^{-1} (top left). (B) The angle is 60° but the sample cursor is not aligned with either the flow or the vessel wall. The resulting velocity is 71.63 cm s^{-1}, 20% less than the velocity determination with the correct alignment.

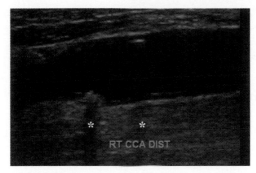

Figure 1.8 Shadowing artifact. The asterisks indicate the region of a shadowing artifact deep in an area of vascular calcification. The decreased echoes deep in the area of calcification are more prominent for the dense calcification on the left.

Artifacts

Errors in acoustic presentation occur because of both anatomic and technical factors. Shadowing occurs distal to dense objects (Figure 1.8). The image is less bright in the region being interrogated by fewer sound waves. In contrast, enhancement of the gray scale occurs distal to echo-free or liquid-filled structures. Multiple reflections from an interface (reverberation) can result in the addition of structures to the image. Refraction of the ultrasound beam can lead to improper placement of the structure on an image, and shadowing at the edge of large structures. Mirror image artifacts are produced when an object is proximal to a highly reflective surface, such as the pleura. Interaction with the reflector alters the timing of the returning echoes. The resulting image display includes a false echo equidistant from the reflector.

Reference list

1 Carroll BA. Carotid ultrasound. Neuroimaging Clin N Am 1996; 6(4):875–897.
2 Tabrizchi R, Pugsley MK. Methods of blood flow measurement in the arterial circulatory system. J Pharmacol Toxicol Methods 2000; 44(2):375–384.
3 Cloutier G, Allard L, Durand LG. Characterization of blood flow turbulence with pulsed-wave and power Doppler ultrasound imaging. J Biomech Eng 1996; 118(3):318–325.
4 Grossman W. Blood flow measurements: the cardiac output and vascular resistance. In: Baim D (ed.), Grossman's Cardiac Catheterization, Angiography, and Intervention, 6th edn., pp. 159–178. Boston: Lippincott Williams & Wilkins, 2000.
5 Cosgrove D, Eckersley R, Blomley M, Harvey C. Quantification of blood flow. Eur Radiol 2001; 11(8):1338–1344.
6 Gorg C, Riera-Knorrenschild J, Dietrich J. Pictorial review: colour Doppler ultrasound flow patterns in the portal venous system. Br J Radiol 2002; 75(899):919–929.
7 Langer SG, Carter SJ, Haynor DR, *et al.* Image acquisition: ultrasound, computed tomography, and magnetic resonance imaging. World J Surg 2001; 25(11):1428–1437.

2 Instrumentation

Michael R. Jaff and Emile R. Mohler III

A wide variety of instruments may be used in the vascular laboratory for the diagnosis of patients with vascular disease. This chapter reviews the technical aspects of commonly used instruments in the vascular laboratory and the methods employed to ensure that optimal images and accurate data are obtained.

Ultrasound physics considerations for optimal imaging

Ultrasound is defined as a high-frequency sound wave which humans cannot hear, with frequencies greater than 20,000 Hz or 20 kHz ($k = 10^3$). Sound waves with a frequency of less than 20 Hz are referred to as infrasound, which humans also cannot hear. Sound occurs as a result of forces on the medium (e.g. air, water, or metal) that are created by forces acting on the molecules, causing them to oscillate about their average position. The motion of molecules is repetitive, and a cycle occurs which can be used to describe this sequence of changes in molecular motion that recurs at regular intervals. Sound cannot occur in a vacuum, but requires an elastic, deformable medium for propagation, such as a gas, liquid, or solid.

The frequency of a sound wave is the number of vibrations that a molecule within the sound wave makes per second or, in other words, the number of times the cycle is repeated per second. The pattern that results from the movement of the particles in the medium across their average position is described in mathematical terms as a "wave." For example, an electronic signal causes a speaker to vibrate or oscillate at the frequency of the sound being produced, which creates the movement of air molecules in a wave pattern. Sound waves are commonly embodied into two types: longitudinal and transverse. The longitudinal wave is one in which the molecules vibrate back and forth in the same direction as the traveling wave. Transverse waves are those moving in a perpendicular direction to the propagation of the wave energy. The wavelength is the distance between two successive density zones and is usually expressed in metric units. Waves traveling through the medium may progress at different speeds, termed the acoustic velocity. This acoustic velocity depends on the density and compressibility of the medium through which the wave is traveling. The diagnostic image from an ultrasound probe is based on the *reflected* rather than the transmitted energy. The interactions of ultrasound with the tissue being examined are similar to those that occur with light, and include reflection, refraction, scattering, defraction, divergence, interference, and absorption. All of these interactions, except for interference, cause a reduction in the intensity of the beam, termed attenuation. Interference may increase or decrease the sound wave intensity.

Optimizing the ultrasound image

The ultrasound probes and definitions of the settings available on ultrasound machines vary according to the vendor, but there are some common probes and settings that are used to optimize the ultrasound image.

Ultrasound probe choice

Different ultrasound systems may provide probes with a spectrum of wavelength capability. The ultrasound wave is produced by passing an electrical current through a piezoelectric crystal. The crystal expands and contracts with the frequency of the electrical signal. The effective radiating area of ultrasound from the transducer is always smaller than the transducer face-plate; therefore, this should be considered on imaging tissue. All transducers can be broadly divided into linear array transducers and curved array transducers. The linear array transducer is a straight line of rectangular elements that produces rectangular images composed of many vertical, parallel scan lines, and is useful for vascular imaging as well as ultrasound-guided procedures, such as access line placement, biopsies, and drainage procedures. The curved array (also known as a convex array) transducer operates similarly to the linear array transducer, but produces a sector image, and is typically used for abdominal imaging. The abdominal aorta and renal arteries are imaged with a curved array transducer. In general, the lower frequency probes, such as those of 3–5 MHz, are used for imaging tissue deeper than 2 cm. More superficial vessels are imaged at higher megahertz values, such as at 8–12 MHz. The high-frequency linear intra-operative probe (10.5 MHz) can be used intra-operatively to image vessels.

The ultrasound wave is most efficiently transmitted to tissue via a conducting medium, such as ultrasound gel. As the ultrasound frequency increases, more energy is absorbed in the tissue. Therefore, ultrasound delivered at lower frequencies tends to travel through superficial tissue and is absorbed at a greater depth. Low-frequency transducers provide greater depth of penetration, but sacrifice image definition. High-frequency transducers provide excellent tissue and image characteristics, but are only effective in superficial imaging.

Another important aspect of ultrasound imaging is the type of tissue being evaluated. Ultrasound is absorbed at different rates by different tissues because of differences in water and protein content. For example, skin and adipose tissue absorb less acoustic energy than muscle, tendon, and ligaments. Bone absorbs the greatest amount of ultrasound energy.

In summary, commercially available ultrasound units generate frequencies of

2–10 million cycles per second (MHz). When an electronic voltage is transmitted to an oscillator, a crystal vibrates and emits an ultrasound beam with a defined frequency in the range of 2–10 MHz. The ultrasound beam hits various targets in its path (i.e. soft tissue, bone, and flowing blood), and is reflected back to the crystal[1].

B mode imaging

Ultrasound units available today use B mode ("brightness") technology to provide a real-time, gray scale image. Duplex ultrasound refers to B mode real-time imaging and focused analysis of the velocity of flowing blood in arteries and veins, i.e. Doppler spectral waveform analysis.

The resolving capability of an ultrasound system depends on the following: (i) the axial/lateral resolution; (ii) the spatial resolution; (iii) the contrast resolution; and (iv) the temporal resolution. The axial resolution specifies how close together two objects can be along the access of the beam, yet still be detected as two separate objects. The frequency (wavelength) affects the axial resolution. The lateral resolution is the ability to resolve two adjacent objects that are perpendicular to the beam axis as separate objects. The beam width affects the lateral resolution. The spatial resolution, also referred to as the detail resolution, is the combination of the axial and lateral resolution. The contrast resolution is the ability to resolve two adjacent objects of similar intensity/reflective properties as separate objects.

Machine settings to optimize ultrasound B mode image

In order to optimize the ultrasound image, there are several adjustments that can be made to enhance the image. Changes to the resolution of the image are commonly referred to as "knobology," and must be mastered for each ultrasound vendor. The three main "knobs" available on most machines include the gain, compression, and depth knobs.

Gain knob

The gain knob can be turned to adjust the brightness of the image. Newer systems may have an automatic gain compensation for imaging. The time gain control (TGC) knobs present on most machines allow for variable gain over the imaging field in the horizontal dimension. Some machines also have gain knobs which allow for variable gain change in the vertical dimension. One of the most common mistakes in ultrasound imaging is the use of incorrect gain settings. Insufficient gain can result in missed structures of low reflectivity, such as thrombi. Excessive gain can result in false echoes or oversaturation, which may obscure important diagnostic image characteristics, such as shadowing or enhancement (Figure 2.1A,B).

Noise caused by excess gain can be resolved by decreasing the overall gain or selecting a different transducer. A low gain artifact can be resolved by increasing the overall gain, increasing the far gain, or applying more acoustic coupling gel.

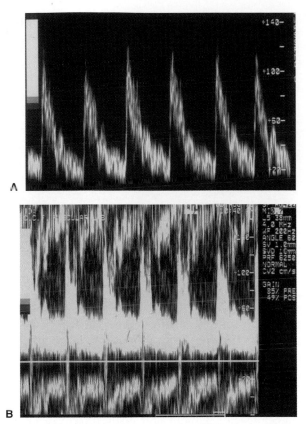

Figure 2.1 (A) Appropriate Doppler gain. (B) Doppler gain set high, causing aliasing and artifactual spectral broadening.

Shadowing caused by the ultrasound beam striking a strong reflective interface (i.e. bony structures, a gallstone, or arterial calcification) may be managed by scanning around the object causing the shadowing (Figure 2.2). A reverberation is caused by sound interfacing with two structures of markedly different acoustic properties. This may be caused by an inadequate amount of gel or obstructing bowel gas. A corrective technique for this problem is to change the angle of the transducer, to apply more gel, or to rotate the patient. An enhancement artifact may be caused by sound traveling through fluid-filled structures without attenuation, e.g. a cyst, commonly seen in renal parenchymal imaging. The enhancement problem may be overcome by reducing the overall gain and decreasing the far gain.

Compression knob

A distinguishing feature of ultrasound images is the oriented "speckled texture" produced by the physics underlying the data acquisition. Owing to its orientation, which changes somewhat across the image, the speckled energy is

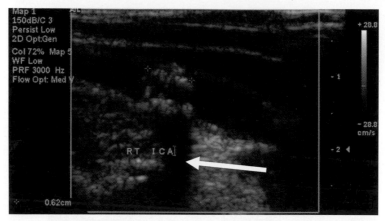

Figure 2.2 Gray scale image of a complex heterogeneous plaque within the proximal internal carotid artery. Note the calcification within the plaque and the associated acoustic shadowing posterior to the plaque (arrow).

typically concentrated in certain regions. The speckle is caused by scattered reflections produced by features that are small with respect to the wavelength. These multiple small reflections result from a rough scattering surface within fine scattering structures. Depending on the context and application, speckle in medical images used for diagnostic purposes may be viewed as a signal or noise. For example, speckle can be used to characterize tissue or can mask important features. A compression algorithm is available on most machines in order to allow for smoother imaging without altering the image in a noticeable way.

Ultrasound compression is also a term used to describe various techniques that allow for the transmission of an image via telemedicine. Some of these include fast Fourier transform, discrete cosine transform, wavelets, quadtrees transform, fractals, histogram thresholding, and run-length coding. The overall purpose of these compressed images is to reduce storage requirements and to make data transmission more convenient. The choice of the correct depth setting is a trade-off between achieving an adequate field of view to resolve all relevant structures and maximizing detail resolution. The depth should be adjusted so that the target vessel or structure is centered in the image.

Depth knob

The depth setting allows for a change in the field of view. The choice of the correct depth setting is a trade-off between achieving an adequate field of view to resolve all relevant structures and maximizing detail resolution. The depth should be adjusted so that the target vessel or structure is centered in the image.

Doppler ultrasound

Christian Doppler described the physics of ultrasonography by identifying the

Doppler shift[2]. Using the velocity of flowing blood, the velocity of sound in tissue, the difference between the frequency of transmitted and reflected sound, and the cosine of the angle of the ultrasound beam to the direction of flowing blood, the velocity of blood in vessels can be measured. This geometric relationship allows ultrasonographers to quantify degrees of stenosis based on the velocity of blood in the various segments of the vessels. Many vascular beds have been studied using duplex ultrasonography. Each arterial system that undergoes duplex interrogation generates ranges of flow velocities which determine degrees of stenosis within the artery.

As a result of the "Doppler" equation, it is clear that the cosine of the angle of the ultrasound beam to flowing blood is critical. Incorrect Doppler angles will result in false Doppler velocities, and therefore in diagnoses which are inaccurate. By convention, the Doppler angle is commonly kept at 60° or less to avoid the overestimation of Doppler velocities (Figure 2.3).

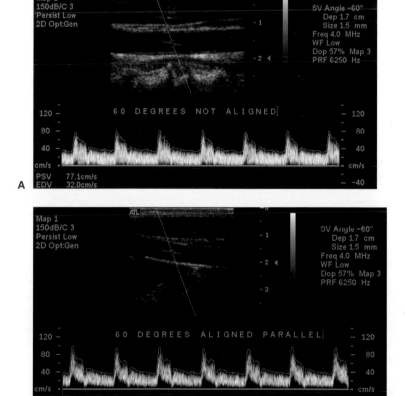

Figure 2.3 (A) Doppler angle is not parallel to the vessel wall. (B) Doppler angle is perfectly aligned and parallel to the vessel wall.

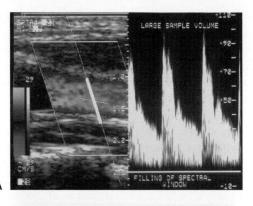

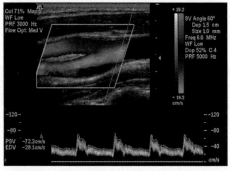

Figure 2.4 (A) Inappropriate sample volume enlargement resulting in artifactual spectral broadening, suggesting a diseased artery. (B) Same artery with accurate, small sample volume, resulting in no spectral broadening in a normal artery.

Spectral broadening is often used to distinguish between completely normal and mildly diseased internal carotid arteries. If the sample volume is inappropriately enlarged, this may result in artifactual spectral broadening. Therefore, all images must use the smallest sample volume possible, unless spectral broadening is not employed as a diagnostic criterion (i.e. renal artery duplex ultrasonography) (Figure 2.4).

Aliasing is a common artifact of Doppler ultrasonography, and must be recognized and corrected for accurate imaging. Aliasing is a static distortion caused by a low pulse repetition frequency (PRF). When the Doppler waveform exceeds the Nyquist limit, aliasing occurs. The Nyquist limit is the maximal measurable frequency, which represents one-half of the sampling frequency of the PRF (Figure 2.5). To resolve aliasing, the PRF should be increased, the baseline lowered, and the depth of field accurately placed.

Color Doppler knob

Color Doppler is a pulse-echo Doppler flow principle that allows for the generation of a color image. This image is superimposed on the two-dimensional image. The red and blue display provides information with regard to the direction and velocity of flow. Regardless of the color, the top of the color bar repre-

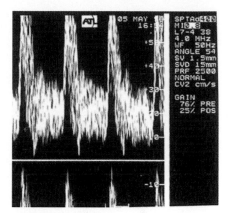

Figure 2.5 Doppler spectrum demonstrating "aliasing," where the pulse repetition frequency is too low, resulting in a "wrap around" of the waveform. This waveform exceeds the Nyquist limit.

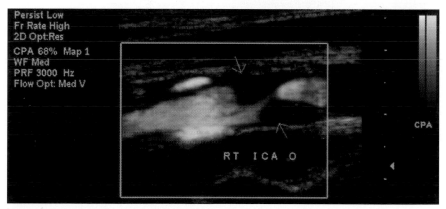

Figure 2.6 Color power angiogram of a severe right internal carotid artery stenosis. Note the marked reduction in luminal caliber at the site of the most severe stenosis. The arrows indicate atherosclerotic plaque.

sents flow coming towards the scan head and the bottom of the bar represents flow away from the scan head.

Power Doppler, or power angiography, is generated from flow information based on the amplitude or strength of the blood cell motion (Figure 2.6). It does not provide directional information. Therefore, power Doppler does not display aliasing. Color Doppler provides better sensitivity to slow flow states, such as may occur in a nearly occluded vessel. Power Doppler is also less angle dependent than traditional color Doppler, but more sensitive to motion artifacts.

Reference list

1 Stewart JH, Grubb M. Understanding vascular ultrasonography. Mayo Clin Proc 1992; 67(12):1186–1196.
2 Nelson TR, Pretorius DH. The Doppler signal: where does it come from and what does it mean? Am J Roentgenol 1988; 151(3):439–447.

PART II

II Cerebrovascular

CHAPTER 3

3 Neurosonology

Eric Edward Smith, Karen Lisa Furie,
Ferdinando S. Buonanno, Madhu B. Vijayappa
and J. Philip Kistler

Carotid duplex ultrasound of the extracranial cerebral vasculature and transcranial Doppler ultrasound of the intracranial cerebral circulation, particularly the great vessels at the base of the brain, are uniquely able to assess arterial flow in the major arteries that feed the brain (Figure 3.1A,B). The assessment of cerebral flow is optimized when these techniques are used in combination in a thorough "neurosonology" study. Carotid duplex scanning techniques are described in Chapter 4. Transcranial Doppler uses a low-megahertz (2 MHz) range-gated Doppler probe. When the probe is placed over the eye (transorbital approach), flow in the ophthalmic artery and intracranial (siphon) portion of the internal carotid artery can be insonated (Figure 3.1). When the probe is placed on the temporal bone window, the proximal portions of the middle, anterior, and posterior cerebral arteries can be insonated. Positioning the probe at the occipital–cervical junction (foramen magnum approach) permits an evaluation of the distal vertebral arteries and the basilar artery. The standard depths of insonation are presented in Figure 3.2.

In this chapter, the four major applications of neurosonology are discussed: (i) ischemic cerebrovascular disease; (ii) intracranial hemorrhage; (iii) intensive care monitoring; and (iv) other diagnostic applications.

Ischemic cerebrovascular disease

Unlike ischemic coronary disease, ischemic cerebrovascular disease [transient ischemic attack (TIA) or stroke] has several prominent causes other than atherothrombosis. When considering endarterectomy or stenting of the internal carotid artery, these other potential causes must be evaluated to ensure that appropriate stroke prevention interventions are initiated[1]. Ischemic cerebrovascular disease has four main causes as outlined by the National Institutes of Health (NIH) Stroke Databank[2]: atherothrombotic disease (15%), small vessel lacunar disease (25%), other rarer causes including dissection of the internal carotid artery and the vertebral artery (3%), and cerebral embolism from the aortic arch, heart, or unknown source (60%)[2]. In each of these ischemic TIA or stroke subtypes, the application of neurosonology is vital to the stroke neurologist. This is not only true in acute stroke care management, but also in making decisions

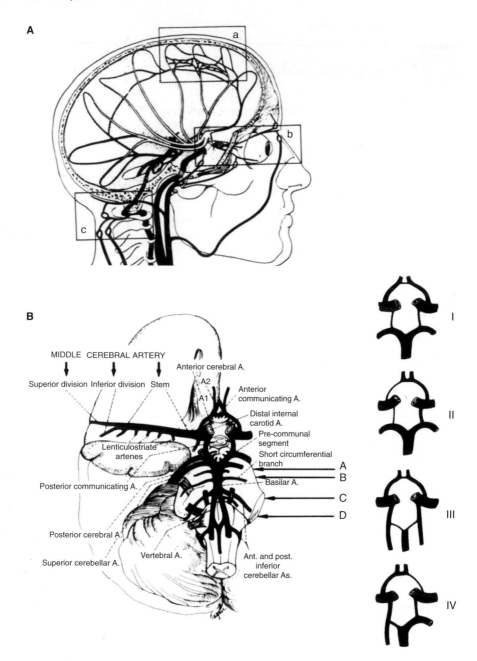

about procedures to deal with atherothrombotic disease, i.e. endarterectomy and/or stenting. Neurosonology is especially useful for following patients with large vessel atherothrombotic disease and dissection over time to document the progression or regression of disease and the effectiveness of preventative

Figure 3.1 (A) Arrangement of the major arteries of the right side carrying blood from the heart to the brain. Also shown are vessels of the collateral circulation that may modify the effects of cerebral ischemia (a, b, c). Not shown is the circle of Willis, which also provides a source for the collateral circulation. a, The anastomotic channels between the distal branches of the anterior and middle cerebral arteries, termed border zone or watershed anastomotic channels. Note that they also occur between the posterior and middle cerebral arteries and between the anterior and posterior cerebral arteries. b, Anastomotic channels occurring through the orbit between branches of the external carotid artery and the ophthalmic branch of the internal carotid artery. c, Wholly extracranial anastomotic channels between the muscular branches of the ascending cervical arteries and muscular branches of the occipital artery that anastomose with the distal cerebral artery. Note that the occipital artery arises from the external carotid artery, thereby allowing reconstitution of flow in the vertebral artery from the carotid circulation. (Courtesy of C. M. Fisher, MD.) (B) Diagram (transect) of the brainstem, cerebellum, inferior right frontal lobe, and temporal lobe. The principal branches of the vertebral basilar arterial system are shown. Small branches of the vertebral and basilar arteries that penetrate the medulla and pons are not shown. The stem of the middle cerebral artery with its small, deep, penetrating branches is shown. Roman numerals I, II, III, and IV represent some of the possible variations of the circle of Willis as a result of atresia of one or more of its arterial components. (Courtesy of C. M. Fisher, MD.)

therapies[3–5]. In this section, each of the four TIA and ischemic stroke subtypes is discussed with regard to the application of neurosonology techniques.

Large vessel atherothrombotic disease — extra- and intracranial (15%)[2]

Just as in the heart and kidneys, and the extremities, large vessel extra- and intracranial atherothrombotic disease has a predilection for specific focal sites. The origin of the internal carotid artery, i.e. bifurcation of the common carotid artery, makes up two-thirds of cases and three intracranial sites make up one-third. The intracranial sites include the siphon portion of the internal carotid artery, the middle cerebral artery stem, and the vertebrobasilar junction. At each of these sites, ischemic cerebrovascular disease, either TIA or stroke, is caused by thrombus formation and embolism (artery-to-artery embolism) or by increasing stenosis limiting the flow distally and signaled by lower perfusion, i.e. low-flow ischemic TIA or stroke. At the origin of the internal carotid artery, artery-to-artery embolism is the most common cause. Low-flow TIA or stroke occurs only when the atherothrombotic lesion narrows the vessel to > 70% stenosis, producing a pressure drop across the lesion as a result of inadequate collateral flow through the ophthalmic circulation or circle of Willis[4,5]. Neurosonology is applied to these four sites as outlined below.

Bifurcation at the origin of the internal carotid artery/bifurcation of the common carotid artery

At this site, an atheromatous plaque occurs most often in the posterior surface near the vertebral body, i.e. at the origin of the internal carotid artery. Increases in the peak systolic and end-diastolic velocity, as well as in the carotid index, have reliably provided highly sensitive criteria for the detection of these lesions. Recently, eight 100%-specific criteria have been developed for the identification

Vessel	Window	Direction	Depth (mm)
M1	Transtemporal	Toward	50–65
M2	Transtemporal	Away > Toward	35–45
A1	Transtemporal	Away	55–80
TICA	Transtemporal	Toward	55–75
P1	Transtemporal	Toward	55–80
P2	Transtemporal	Away	55–70
OA	Transorbital	Toward	40–50
Siphon	Transorbital	Away, Toward[1]	55–70
VA	Suboccipital	Away	55–75
BA	Suboccipital	Away	85–120
ECICA	Submental	Away	45–50

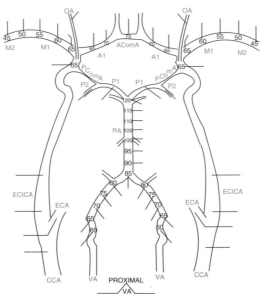

Figure 3.2 Schematic diagram of the extra- and intracranial arteries. The range-gated pulse Doppler depths of insonation are displayed for anterior and posterior transcranial Doppler. Extracranial carotid duplex insonates the mid-common carotid artery (CCA) and the CCA bifurcation into the extracranial internal carotid artery (EICA) and external carotid artery (ECA), as well as the mid-neck portion of the extracranial vertebral artery. Anterior transcranial Doppler insonates the ophthalmic artery (OA), the siphon portion of the distal internal carotid artery (ICA), the middle cerebral artery stem (M1) and its bifurcation (M2), the anterior cerebral artery stem (A1), and the posterior cerebral artery stem (P1). Posterior transcranial Doppler insonates the distal intracranial portion of the vertebral artery (VA) and the basilar artery (BA).

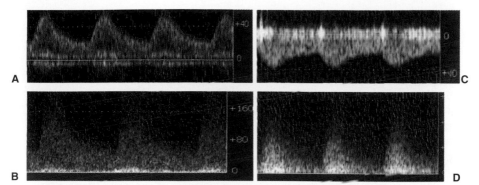

Figure 3.3 Common spectral patterns noted by transcranial Doppler. (A) Normal flow (intracranial capacitance artery). (B) Low-resistance flow (slow systolic upstroke with long diastolic runoff and low pulse pressure) (C) Attenuated flow (distal arterial obstructive lesion). (D) Streamlined flow with turbulence (high-speed jet at the point of arterial stenosis with turbulent or disturbed flow immediately distal to it).

Table 3.1 Carotid Doppler criteria to determine residual lumen ≤1.5 mm

	Sensitivity	Specificity	PPV	NPV	Accuracy
PSV >220	99	26	82	86	82
PSV >360	85	78	93	62	82
PSV >440	58	100	100	42	68
EDV >115	82	70	90	53	79
EDV >155	63	100	100	45	72
Carotid index >3.5	99	35	83	89	84
Carotid index >5.5	80	78	94	53	80
Carotid index >10	30	100	100	30	46
PSV >440 or EDV >130 or carotid index >9	82	87	95	59	83
Highly specific criteria: PSV >440 or EDV >155 or carotid index >10	72	100	100	52	79
Highly sensitive criteria: PSV >200 and (EDV >140 or carotid index >4.5)	96	61	89	82	88

PPV, positive predictive value; NPV, negative predictive value. PSV and EDV values are centimeters per second.

of a lesion severe enough to be associated with a pressure drop across it, i.e. >70% stenosis[4,5] (Figure 3.3). Although alone, each of these highly specific criteria is not highly sensitive, when combined, the sensitivity is also highly acceptable, i.e. >80%. The criteria are based on the actual pathologic assessment of the intact endarterectomy specimen and are noted in Table 3.1. The peak velocities are more sensitive than the mean velocity to these criteria, and are therefore used for intracranial vasculature assessment. The criteria assess the adequacy of collateral flow to the ipsilateral hemisphere above the stenosis through the extracranial ophthalmic vasculature and the circle of Willis (Figures 3.1A,B & 3.2). Although B mode ultrasound imaging and newer research techniques offer promise for the identification of the characteristics of the atherothrombotic plaque, particularly whether or not it is actively progressing or whether a thrombus is involved, currently the highly sensitive but nonspecific velocity criteria of Strandis *et al.*[3] and the highly specific criteria[4,5] are commonly used to detect progression. Importantly, the transcranial Doppler flow spectrum in the middle cerebral artery stem can provide information about the adequacy of collateral flow distal to a hemodynamically significant carotid stenosis. Low-resistance patterns with a low pulse pressure and a slow upstroke in systole (Figure 3.3B) are suggestive of a proximal stenosis. The velocity of flow across the circle of Willis from the contralateral A1 anterior cerebral artery through the ipsilateral A1 anterior cerebral artery is also suggestive, particularly with delays in change with breath holding. However, these characteristics are not specific because of the variability of the circle itself (Figure 3.1B).

Siphon portion of the internal carotid artery

Flow by anterior transcranial Doppler analysis of the middle and anterior cerebral flow or flow in the siphon portion of the internal carotid artery or ophthalmic artery changes only if the lesion is hemodynamically significant, i.e. >70% stenosis, and there is a pressure drop across it. Similarly, flow spectra and peak systolic and end-diastolic velocities at the origin of the internal carotid artery change only when the siphon stenosis is hemodynamically significant. An attenuated (blunted or humped) flow spectrum (Figure 3.3C) at the origin of the internal carotid artery, with little diastolic flow, is indicative of a more distal (hemodynamically significant) carotid lesion, particularly when there is minimal plaque formation at the origin of the internal carotid artery. A low-resistance flow spectrum (Figure 3.3B) in the middle cerebral and anterior cerebral stem, with high-flow-velocity collateralization across the anterior circle of Willis, is indicative of the same distal internal carotid artery lesion provided that the origin of the internal carotid artery does not have a hemodynamically significant stenosis and the circle of Willis is inadequate to provide sufficient collateral flow.

Atherothrombotic disease of the middle cerebral stem

A stenosis of the middle cerebral artery is detectable when it becomes hemodynamically significant and impedes flow, producing an attenuated flow spectrum (Figure 3.3C) proximal to it. A very high peak systolic velocity with a high end-diastolic flow pattern is indicative of the jet of streamlined flow through the stenosis with turbulence just after the stenotic segment (Figure 3.3D). Occasionally, high velocity in the contralateral A1 anterior cerebral artery can be suggestive of ischemia in the contralateral hemisphere caused by a middle cerebral artery stem stenosis. Blood flows across the anterior communicating artery and up the ipsilateral A2 anterior cerebral artery, and then out over the hemisphere through pial branches to provide cortical surface collateral to the middle cerebral artery territory.

Atherothrombotic disease at the vertebrobasilar junction

The extracranial carotid duplex study may show some attenuation of flow in the vertebral artery. More commonly, if the stenotic lesion is in the distal vertebral artery, transcranial Doppler may detect high-velocity streamlined flow (Figure 3.3D) distal to the stenosis. With mid-basilar atherothrombotic lesions, the atherothrombotic stenosis will increase the peak systolic and end-diastolic flow velocities (Figure 3.3D), but the velocities of flow distally and proximally will be attenuated (Figure 3.3C). Severely stenotic or occlusive lesions of the proximal basilar or bilateral vertebral arteries can result in the reversal of flow in the basilar artery if the posterior communicating arteries provide adequate collateral flow from the intracranial internal carotid arteries.

Rare sites of atherothrombotic disease

These sites include the more distal segments of the anterior, middle, and posterior cerebral arteries, the origins of the larger vessels coming off the basilar artery, and the origins of the great vessels. Transcranial Doppler cannot directly insonate these vessels, but there may be indirect evidence of disease at these intracranial sites if the lesion is severe enough to affect the spectrum in the basilar artery or middle or posterior cerebral arteries.

Small vessel lacunar disease (25%)[2]

Small vessel disease, by definition, is the occlusion of a single penetrating vessel that comes off the circle of Willis, the basilar artery, the distal vertebral (intracranial portion) artery, or the middle cerebral artery stem. The single vessel occlusion definition of a lacunar stroke was proven through serial section of the brain at post-mortem[6]. Lacunae have a finite size and occur in the pons (penetrating branches of the basilar artery), in the basal ganglion area (penetrating branches of the middle cerebral stem) and in the thalamus (penetrating branches of the posterior cerebral artery). The vessels that are occluded are between 200 and 800 μm in diameter. The occlusive pathology most often is lipohyalinosis and, less often, atheroma at the origin of the penetrating vessel. Although transcranial Doppler assessment of flow is not possible in these vessels, normal flow should be detected in the parent vessel from which they arise, i.e. the basilar artery, the middle cerebral stem, or the posterior cerebral stem. If not, the clinical syndrome may represent pathology in the parent vessel that could lead to devastating worsening.

Other, including carotid and vertebral artery dissection (3%)[2]

Dissection of the internal carotid artery and of the vertebral artery occurs at the junction at which they interface with the petrous bone and the foramen transversarum, respectively[7]. In contrast with atherosclerotic narrowing, dissections do not commonly originate at the origin of the internal carotid artery, at the origin of the vertebral artery, or in the intracranial large arteries. Dissection may extend to the internal carotid artery origin or the vertebral artery origin, thereby blocking them at the origin. Alternatively, lesions can dissect up into the intracranial portion of the distal internal carotid artery and into the middle cerebral stem, or into the distal vertebral artery and up into the basilar artery. The artery may occlude at any site to which the dissection extends. Artery-to-artery embolism, however, is the most common cause of ischemic stroke or TIA. With this pathophysiology in mind, neurosonology is useful in the following ways. First, if a dissection of the internal carotid artery impedes flow in the carotid artery, it can be detected by an attenuated flow spectrum (Figure 3.3C) at the origin of the internal carotid artery. If it does not, carotid artery duplex should be normal. Secondly, impedance of flow in the dissected internal carotid artery can be inferred through changes in flow patterns in the circle of Willis or through the orbit. Specifically, collateralization towards the ipsilateral middle cerebral stem is noted by increased velocity in the contralateral A1 segment of the anterior cerebral artery and by abnormal (low-resistance) (Figure 3.3B) flow in the middle cerebral stem if the circle of Willis is atretic. Blockage of the middle cerebral artery stem by embolism from carotid dissection can also occur and be detected by a highly impeded (attenuated) flow spectrum in the middle cerebral artery stem.

Vertebral artery dissections are suggested by an attenuation of the flow in the proximal or distal vertebral artery (Figure 3.3C), but this finding may not be present. The important point is that normal flow in the vertebral or basilar artery, the carotid artery, the circle of Willis, or the ipsilateral middle cerebral stem does not rule out dissection of the vertebral or carotid artery. Neurosonology is useful in following the course of a dissection, particularly as the clot absorbs and the dissection stenosis improves.

Cerebral embolism from the aortic arch, heart, or unknown source (60%)[2]

Cerebral emboli from each of these three sources (aortic arch, heart, or unknown) are largely composed of thrombus. Less often, the embolic material is atheromatous or fibrotic debris. The thrombotic portion of an embolus generally lyses spontaneously. This process may be augmented by fibrinolytic therapies. Emboli migrate as they lyse and disperse. Embolic stroke occurs when lysis does not occur soon enough and blood flow to the appropriate arterial territory is impeded long enough to cause infarction. Transient cerebral ischemia due to emboli occurs when lysis takes place early and/or there is adequate collateral flow to prevent distal flow reduction.

Transcranial Doppler assessment of cerebral embolism is extremely important. Most importantly, it documents instantaneously whether or not the embolic fragment has migrated and lysed in the vessel suspected of producing the ischemia, usually the basilar or middle cerebral artery stem. The immediate detection of nonlysed emboli in the distal vertebral arteries, basilar artery (posterior transcranial Doppler), or distal internal carotid artery, middle cerebral artery stem, anterior cerebral artery stem, or posterior cerebral artery stem (anterior transcranial Doppler) has highly important therapeutic implications. If, by transcranial Doppler, the flow patterns are normal in these vessels, it can be assumed that the embolic fragment has migrated and lysed out of the vessel. The improvement of flow in the embolized artery at the base of the brain from an attenuated spectral pattern (Figure 3.3C) to a more normal spectral flow (Figure 3.3A) is highly suggestive of such migration and lysis. The calculation of the risk–benefit of thrombolytic therapy to improve intracerebral flow rests on this point. In addition, it is useful in planning whether or not, in the subacute phase, antithrombotic therapy should be considered to prevent clot propagation. Lastly, there is evidence emerging that ultrasonic techniques aimed directly at the embolic fragment in the vessel at the base of the brain can be beneficial in promoting lysis[8]. Transcranial Doppler modalities may therefore become very important therapeutically, as well as diagnostically, particularly if there is no increased risk of symptomatic hemorrhage into the infarct.

Subarachnoid hemorrhage

The major cause of secondary morbidity following aneurysmal subarachnoid hemorrhage (SAH) is cerebral ischemia as a result of arterial vasospasm. The incidence of *radiographic vasospasm* peaks on the sixth to eighth day following rupture of the aneurysm, and can be detected on catheter angiography in up to 70% of patients on the seventh day. However, the incidence of delayed ischemic neurologic deficits (DINDs) caused by vasospasm is considerably lower at 20–30%, presumably due to adequate collateral supply in many patients. As the major risk factor for vasospasm is the presence of blood and its breakdown products in close proximity to the surface of major cerebral arteries, the vessel segments most likely to be involved are those of the major branches of the circle of Willis at the base of the brain. These are the same vessel segments that can be insonated by transcranial Doppler and, as a result, it has a well-established role in the diagnosis and monitoring of vasospasm[9].

Vasospasm appears on transcranial Doppler as elevations of the peak and mean flow velocities, often in association with evidence of turbulent flow, which may appear as a loss of the normal spectral window. Elevations in flow velocities parallel the known time course of the prevalence of vasospasm, tending to peak approximately 1 week following aneurysm rupture, and then declining to the normal range over the following 1–2 weeks. In contrast with atherosclerotic arterial narrowing, flow velocity elevations in vasospasm are more diffuse (i.e. occur over a longer portion of the arterial segment) and are often paralleled by milder elevations in other arteries or other segments of the same artery. The most severe vasospasm is often detected in the vessel with the closest proximity to the aneurysm, but more remote vessels, even on the contralateral side, may be affected.

Transcranial Doppler velocities correlate well with the presence of radiographic vasospasm (as defined by catheter angiography), less well with cerebral blood flow [as measured by single photon emission computed tomography (SPECT) or other methods], and, not surprisingly, least well with the presence or absence of DINDs. For the middle cerebral artery, a mean flow velocity of > 120 cm s^{-1} has been cited in the literature as indicative of the presence of vasospasm. Increasing the cut-off to > 200 cm s^{-1} increases the specificity but significantly lowers the sensitivity. If vasospasm progresses and becomes very severe, flow velocities may ultimately decrease as a result of limitation of the flow volume. A recent meta-analysis pooled the results from all methodologi-

Table 3.2 Sensitivity and specificity for vasospasm due to aneurysmal subarachnoid hemorrhage[10].

Artery	Number of pooled subjects	Criteria for presence of vasospasm (mean flow velocity) (cm s^{-1})	Sensitivity (%)	Specificity (%)
Middle cerebral artery	198	> 120	67	99
Intracranial internal carotid artery	84	> 90	25	91
Anterior cerebral artery	108	> 120	42	76
Posterior cerebral artery	47	> 90	48	69
Basilar artery	42	> 60	77	79
Vertebral artery	42	> 60	44	88

All methodologically robust studies prior to 1998 were included. The results are based on a single study, except for the middle cerebral artery (five studies) and anterior cerebral artery (three studies).

cally robust studies to determine the sensitivity and specificity for vasospasm in each artery[10]. A relatively high sensitivity was shown in the middle cerebral artery and basilar artery, while a lower sensitivity was seen in the anterior cerebral artery, intracranial internal carotid artery, posterior cerebral artery, and vertebral artery (Table 3.2). This variability in sensitivity is probably a result of technical factors related to specific vessel anatomy, such as the angle of the vessel in relation to the Doppler probe, as well as the overall difficulty of insonation.

The imperfect correlation between the transcranial Doppler velocity and the degree of angiographic vasospasm is understandable when the complex nature of vasospasm is considered. As vasospasm is a multifocal disease, it may be present *at* the insonation site, *proximal* to the site, *distal* to the site, or in some combination. In addition, studies have suggested that some patients with SAH may have the uncoupling of blood flow from neuronal metabolism (i.e. impaired autoregulation) with resultant hyperemia. The influence of systemic factors must also be considered when interpreting abnormal transcranial Doppler results. The elevation of the mean flow velocity not due to vasospasm (i.e. false positives) may occur with induced hypertension (a commonly used treatment for vasospasm and DIND), other hyperdynamic cardiovascular states, fever, anemia, hypercarbia, post-surgical vessel stenosis due to clip placement, or when the insonated vessel serves as a channel for collateral flow or an adjacent vessel in vasospasm is inadvertently insonated. In addition, the influence of systemic factors may be increased when there is impaired autoregulation. To account for the influence of systemic hemodynamic factors and impaired autoregulation, Lindegaard proposed the calculation of the ratio of the middle cerebral artery mean flow velocity to the ipsilateral extracranial internal carotid artery mean flow velocity (insonated at a depth of 50 mm with the probe below the angle of the jaw and directed superiorly); values of < 3.0 are very uncommon in vasospasm, while values of > 6.0 are highly specific for vasospasm[11].

It should also be noted that false negative results may occur. As transcranial Doppler is performed without direct visualization of the vessel, a higher than expected Doppler angle cannot be corrected and may lead to a significant underestimation of the true velocity. Proximal stenosis, low cardiac output, coexisting raised intracranial pressure (ICP) with a reduction in cerebral blood flow, operator inexperience, or the presence of vasospasm in distal vessels that cannot be insonated by transcranial Doppler may also cause false negatives. If a clinical syndrome consistent with DIND is present, despite nondiagnostic transcranial Doppler findings, the presence of vasospasm should still be considered.

Frequent screening with transcranial Doppler may allow the early diagnosis of vasospasm, which often precedes DIND by 1–2 days, allowing high-risk patients to be targeted for additional therapies, such as catheter angioplasty or administration of intra-arterial vasodilators. A 24 h velocity increase of greater than 50 cm s^{-1} may also be associated with an increased risk of subsequent brain hypoperfusion due to vasospasm. In our neurointensive care unit, baseline transcranial Doppler is obtained during the first 24 h of admission and daily transcranial Doppler is continued until the high-risk period has passed.

Other intracranial hemorrhage

Transcranial Doppler has a limited role in the diagnosis and management of intracranial bleeding other than SAH. Nonspecific signs of raised ICP, described below, may be detected. One study of primary intracerebral hemorrhage found that elevation of the pulsatility index (Figure 3.4) to greater than 1.75, probably reflecting increased vascular resistance as a result of significantly increased ICP, predicted the 30 day mortality with 80% sensitivity and 94% specificity[12]. If an arteriovenous malformation is present, the pulsatility index may be low in the feeding arteries, consistent with reduced resistance to blood flow as a result of direct arteriovenous shunting; however, transcranial Doppler cannot be considered a sensitive test for the detection of vascular malformations.

Intensive care monitoring

Raised intracranial pressure

The initial transcranial Doppler sign of increasing ICP is an increase in the pulsatility index, consistent with a global increase in the distal vascular resistance (Figure 3.5). This change may be seen even at a stage at which the cerebral perfusion pressure and cerebral blood flow are adequate to maintain normal neuronal metabolism and hence normal brain function. However, if ICP continues to increase, the cerebrovascular resistance will continue to increase, ultimately leading to a decrease in the cerebral perfusion pressure and decreased cerebral blood flow. On transcranial Doppler, this is detected as a decline in the mean flow velocity. As ICP approaches diastolic blood pressure, the end-diastolic flow velocity approaches zero and, when ICP exceeds the diastolic blood pressure, there may be reversal of flow with negative diastolic flow velocities. The

$$\text{Pulsatility index} = \frac{\text{(Peak systolic velocity} - \text{End diastolic velocity)}}{\text{(Mean flow velocity)}}$$

Figure 3.4 The pulsatility index is sensitive to the shape of the transcranial Doppler waveform. Normal values range from 0.5 to 1.4. Elevated values are seen in conditions in which there is increased distal resistance to flow.

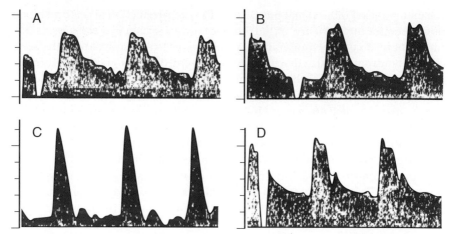

Figure 3.5 Raised intracranial pressure. Baseline MCA recording was normal in a 58-year-old patient with subarachnoid hemorrhage (A). Mild increased ICP developed due to hydrocephalus; repeat MCA recording shows a mild increase in the pulsatility index (PI = 1.2) (B). Following further increase in ICP, MCA recording shows a marked increase in the pulsatility index (PI = 2.1) with minimal diastolic flow (C). After treatment of hydrocephalus and lowering of ICP, MCA recording shows improved diastolic flow and a decrease in the pulsatility index (PI = 1.1) (D). (Courtesy of Raul Nogueira, MD, and Ferdinando Buonanno, MD).

latter pattern is associated with a severe reduction in cerebral blood flow or absent net forward flow and, if persistent and global, it is indicative of cerebrocirculatory arrest and brain death (see below).

There has been interest in the use of transcranial Doppler information to noninvasively estimate ICP. If perfected, transcranial Doppler estimation of ICP could obviate the need for invasive monitoring, or be used as a substitute for invasive monitoring where contraindications, such as the presence of coagulopathy, are present. Several authors have described equations that use characteristics of the middle cerebral artery waveform and systemic arterial waveform to estimate ICP. These estimates correlate reasonably well with invasive measurements by an ICP monitor and are sensitive to changes in ICP or systemic arterial pressure. However, it is likely that the ICP estimates are also dependent on the degree of vasomotor tone, integrity of autoregulation, and possibly the presence or absence of intrinsic vascular pathologies, such as stenosis or vasospasm. Therefore, these methods have not been sufficiently validated to be considered as alternatives to conventional ICP monitoring.

Traumatic brain injury

Patients with traumatic brain injury often have disordered cerebral perfusion as a result of increased ICP and abnormal cerebrovascular autoregulation. Transcranial Doppler signs of raised ICP may be present (see above). Abnormal autoregulation has been demonstrated by evaluating the response of the middle cerebral artery flow velocity to physiologic fluctuations in arterial blood pressure or manipulations of arterial blood pressure or P_{CO_2}. However, studies have

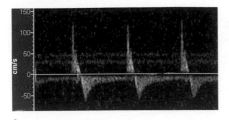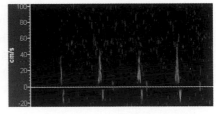

A   **B**

Figure 3.6 Transcranial Doppler patterns consistent with intracranial circulatory arrest and brain death. (A) Oscillatory flow, with a sharp systolic peak followed by a reversal of flow in diastole, indicative of minimal or no net forward flow. (B) Small early systolic spikes of < 200 ms in duration and < 50 cm s^{-1} peak velocity. Intracranial circulatory arrest may also produce absent flow (not depicted).

Table 3.3 World Federation of Neurology criteria for transcranial Doppler diagnosis of brain death[14].

1 Presence of oscillating flow or narrow systolic spikes (see text for description) in all recorded arteries in the anterior and posterior circulation
2 A recording is made from each hemisphere
3 The intracranial diagnosis is confirmed by extracranial bilateral recording of the common carotid artery, internal carotid artery, and vertebral artery
4 If a signal is absent, the diagnosis can still be made if:
   (a) waveforms were present on a prior study, therefore demonstrating that adequate windows for insonation are present; and
   (b) presence of typical extracranial Doppler findings
5 Findings consistent with brain death are documented on two examinations at least 30 min apart
6 Ventricular drains or large openings of the skull, such as decompressive craniectomy, which may interfere with the development of raised intracranial pressure, are not present

failed to find a strong relationship between the loss of autoregulation and long-term outcome. Delayed vasospasm and DIND have been seen in some patients following traumatic brain injury; in comparison with aneurysmal SAH, the incidence appears to be much lower. When DIND is suspected, transcranial Doppler may be used to screen for the presence of vasospasm, as described above.

Brain death
The use of transcranial Doppler as an adjunctive test for brain death is supported by a guideline statement from the American Academy of Neurology[13]. Brain death can be confirmed by the demonstration of net zero flow velocity or minimal flow velocity that is inadequate for neuronal survival; this appears as either narrow systolic peaks followed by negative diastolic flow velocity or small early systolic spikes, defined as a systolic waveform with a duration of < 200 ms and a maximal velocity of < 50 cm s^{-1} (Figure 3.6). These patterns must be present in all insonated intracranial arteries to make the diagnosis. Ultimately, there may be loss of all signal; however, the absence of flow velocities does not, by itself, con-

firm brain death, as some patients may have inadequate temporal windows for insonation. The reported specificity is 97–100% and the sensitivity is 91–100%[13]. The few reported false positives have been patients with some minimal regional arterial flow on catheter angiography, but ultimately all these patients progressed to brain death[14]. In addition, it should be noted that transcranial Doppler findings consistent with brain death can be transiently present immediately following cardiac arrest or during brief severe ICP elevation, such as could occur during re-rupture of a cerebral aneurysm. However, there have been no reported cases of survival when transcranial Doppler signs of circulatory arrest are persistent. A consensus statement from the World Federation of Neurology[14] suggested criteria for a positive study (Table 3.3).

Reference list

1 Kistler JP, Furie KL. Carotid endarterectomy revisited (editorial). N Engl J Med 2000; 342:1743–1744.

2 Sacco RL, Ellenberg JH, Mohr JP, et al. Infarcts of undetermined cause: the NINCDS Stroke Data Bank. Ann Neurol 1989; 25:382–390.

3 Strandis NI, Reutern G-M, Budingen HJ. Ultraschalldiagnostik der Hirnversorgenden Arterien. Stuttgart: Georg Thieme Verlag, 1989.

4 Suwanwela N, Can U, Furie KL, et al. Carotid Doppler ultrasound criteria for internal carotid artery stenosis based on residual lumen diameter calculated from en bloc carotid endarterectomy specimens. Stroke 1996; 27:1965–1969.

5 Can U, Furie KL, Suwanwela N, et al. Transcranial Doppler ultrasound criteria for hemodynamically significant internal carotid artery stenosis based on residual lumen diameter calculated from en bloc endarterectomy specimens. Stroke 1997; 28:1966–1971.

6 Fisher CM. Lacunar strokes and infarcts: a review. Neurology 1982; 32:871–876.

7 Fisher CM, Ojemann RG, Roberson GH. Spontaneous dissection of cervico-cerebral arteries. Can J Neurol Sci 1978; 5(1):9–19.

8 Alexandrov AV. Ultrasound-enhanced thrombolysis for stroke: clinical significance. Eur J Ultrasound 2002; 16:131–140.

9 Sloan MA, Alexandrov AV, Tegeler CH, et al. Assessment: transcranial Doppler ultrasonography: report of the Therapeutics and Technology Assessment Subcommittee of the American Academy of Neurology. Neurology 2004; 62(9):1468–1481.

10 Lysakowski C, Walder B, Costanza MC, Tramer MR. Transcranial Doppler versus angiography in patients with vasospasm due to a ruptured cerebral aneurysm: a systematic review. Stroke 2001; 32(10):2292–2298.

11 Lindegaard KF. The role of transcranial Doppler in the management of patients with subarachnoid haemorrhage—a review. Acta Neurochir Suppl 1999; 72:59–71.

12 Marti-Fabregas J, Belvis R, Guardia E, et al. Prognostic value of Pulsatility Index in acute intracerebral hemorrhage. Neurology 2003; 61(8):1051–1056.

13 Practice parameters for determining brain death in adults (summary statement). The Quality Standards Subcommittee of the American Academy of Neurology. Neurology 1995; 45(5):1012–1014.

14 Ducrocq X, Hassler W, Moritake K, et al. Consensus opinion on diagnosis of cerebral circulatory arrest using Doppler-sonography: Task Force Group on cerebral death of the Neurosonology Research Group of the World Federation of Neurology. J Neurol Sci 1998; 159(2):145–150.

4 Extracranial Carotid and Vertebral Artery Evaluation

Marie Gerhard-Herman

Evaluation of the extracranial carotid arteries

Evaluation of the extracranial carotid arteries provides information on stroke risk and overall cardiovascular risk. Infarction of brain tissue (stroke) occurs when blood flow is occluded to a portion of the brain. These ischemic strokes account for up to 75% of all strokes. Proximal internal carotid artery (ICA) occlusion causes approximately 5% of ischemic strokes. Stroke results in neurologic deficit attributable to a region of the brain with a distinct and specific arterial supply. For example, sudden weakness of one side of the body is attributable to interruption of the contralateral middle cerebral artery supply. The symptoms of vertigo, ataxia, and paresthesia are attributable to interruption of the posterior cerebral artery circulation. Stroke occurs when the lack of blood supply results in brain cell death. The clinical presentation is labeled transient ischemic attack (TIA) if the blood supply is restored within a day, symptoms disappear, and brain cell death does not occur.

The risk of stroke increases with increasing plaque size and with increasing degrees of carotid stenosis. Stroke attributable to ICA stenosis results from atheroemboli originating in the cervical ICA much more often than from insufficient perfusion attributable to high-grade stenosis. The prevalence of ICA atherosclerosis increases with age and with the number of cardiovascular risk factors[1-4]. The presence of carotid atherosclerosis is also a marker for systemic atherosclerosis and is associated with increased cardiovascular risk[5]. For this reason, the Adult Treatment Panel III guidelines identify greater than 50% ICA stenosis as a "coronary heart disease equivalent."

Duplex ultrasound of the carotid arteries is always performed in the clinical setting with a specific query in mind. This query ranges from identifying the cause of a bruit to evaluating ICA stenosis in a patient with TIA.

Anatomy of the neck arteries

Duplex ultrasound examination identifies the carotid and vertebral arteries. The right common carotid artery (CCA) and right subclavian artery originate from the innominate (brachiocephalic) artery, while the left CCA arises directly

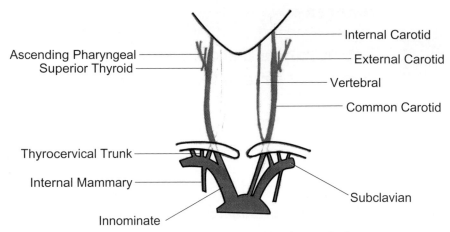

Internal Carotid

Ascending Pharyngeal

Superior Thyroid

External Carotid

Vertebral

Common Carotid

Thyrocervical Trunk

Internal Mammary

Subclavian

Innominate

Figure 4.1 The neck arteries relevant to extracranial carotid duplex examination.

from the aorta (Figure 4.1). Therefore, the origin of the right CCA can be evaluated by ultrasound, while the origin of the left CCA lies below the clavicle and is not accessible to ultrasound. In the absence of disease, arterial waveforms and artery diameters should be similar when compared between the right and left sides of the neck. The vertebral arteries originate from the subclavian arteries, and are visible to ultrasound evaluation only as they course between the neural foramina of the cervical spine. The CCA divides into the ICA and external carotid artery (ECA) near the upper border of the thyroid cartilage. The carotid bulb is the arterial segment with increased diameter, which begins in the distal CCA and extends into the proximal ICA. The ICA continues into the cranium without branching. The ICA supplies the majority of blood flow into the anterior circulation of the brain. In contrast with the ICA, the ECA has many branches within the neck and typically supplies no blood flow to the brain. In the setting of significant ICA disease, the branches of the ECA can become an important collateral pathway for blood flow to the brain. The blood flow through the ECA increases in this situation, and there may also be further dilation of the arteries providing collateral flow.

Examination technique

The duplex ultrasound examination begins with gray scale, transverse imaging from the clavicle to the angle of the jaw. This scan is used to identify the course of the carotid arteries. Transverse color flow evaluation is useful in evaluating the course of tortuous vessels. If the entire course of the vessel is not evident, new acoustic windows are created by asking the patient to turn towards the probe. The transverse images demonstrate atherosclerotic plaque, which appears as thickened areas of the arterial wall that protrude into the lumen. The majority of plaque is present at the bifurcation of the CCA into the ICA and ECA. The

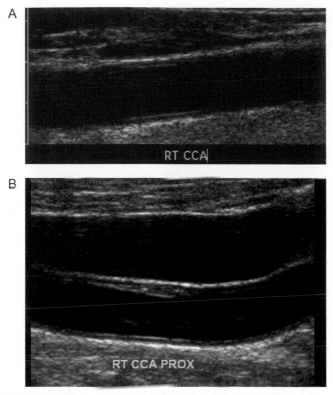

Figure 4.2 Common carotid artery imaged from the anterior (A) and lateral (B) transducer positions.

innermost layers of the artery can be diffusely thickened. This is called intimal medial thickening, and generally precedes overt plaque development. Transverse images are displayed with right and left orientation as though the examiner is looking from the feet with the right side of the body on the left side of the screen.

Ultrasound evaluation is then performed with the transducer rotated longitudinally. The distal artery is displayed on the left side of the screen. The head is typically turned away from the side being scanned. The carotid artery is imaged from both the anterior approach, medial to the sternocleidomastoid muscle, and the lateral approach, through the jugular vein. Directing the ultrasound beam through the jugular vein often results in better elucidation of the anterior wall of the carotid artery. The transducer is kept parallel to the vessel walls to better define the layers of the arterial wall and elucidate the character of the plaque (Figure 4.2). The optimal transducer position is also determined by the patient's anatomy. Thick necks and immobilized cervical spines are two situations in which the transducer position options are limited.

Doppler evaluation

Spectral and color Doppler evaluation is performed with the longitudinal images at a slight angle with respect to the vertical plane. This is accomplished with a slight change in the heel and toe pressure applied to the probe. Spectral Doppler evaluation is made utilizing an angle of 60° between the samples' cursor aligned with the inner arterial wall (or flow jet) and the insonation beam. The sample volume is kept center stream and marched carefully through the CCA and ICA in order to detect the discrete areas of flow abnormality suggestive of stenosis. Forward flow is present throughout the cardiac cycle in the CCA and ICA. Reverse flow in the CCA and ICA is present only in patients with aortic regurgitation, carotid dissection, or distal carotid occlusion.

The spectral Doppler waveform in the CCA is a combination of that found in the ipsilateral ICA and ECA (Figure 4.3A). Reflections, or bumps, in the spectral envelope are evident in younger, healthier individuals with compliant vessels. The ICA feeds the low-resistance bed of the brain, and therefore has prominent diastolic flow indicative of the continuous flow to the brain (Figure 4.3B). Normal peak systolic velocities in the ICA range from 60 to 80 cm s^{-1}. The ECA has antegrade flow with a much smaller diastolic component (Figure 4.3C). It normally supplies the high-resistance arterial beds of the neck and face. A rapid upstroke is evident in all the carotid spectral Doppler waveforms in a normal individual. The ipsilateral ICA and ECA waveforms should look different from each other. Helpful maneuvers in distinguishing ECA and ICA include looking for branches arising from the vessel, and tapping the pre-auricular portion of the temporal artery and looking for deflections in the spectral waveform in the ECA and ICA. The deflections should be clearly evident in the diastolic portion of the ECA waveform. Deflections from tapping the temporal artery are generally not present in the diastolic portion of the ICA waveform. Deflections are rarely seen in the origin of the ICA, and are much less prominent than the deflections from tapping apparent in the ipsilateral ECA.

Color Doppler demonstrates flow separation or reversal in the widened segment of the carotid bulb as a result of the loss of normal laminar flow in this arterial segment. These altered flow characteristics contribute to the development of atherosclerotic plaque at this site in the origin of the ICA.

Figure 4.3 Spectral waveforms in the carotid arteries. (A) The common carotid artery (CCA) waveform is determined in part by the distal flow into the internal carotid artery (ICA) and external carotid artery (ECA). (B) The normal ICA has increased diastolic flow compared with the ECA and CCA. This is a normal low-resistance waveform with a narrow spectrum of velocities. There is normally a clear "spectral window." This region is filled in with lower velocities reflective of turbulence, or when the sample volume is set to encompass the entire diameter of the vessel, including the low velocity at the wall. (C) The ECA has a much lower diastolic flow. The rhythmic deflections seen in the diastolic portion of the second wave are a result of tapping on the ipsilateral temporal artery (branch of the ECA).

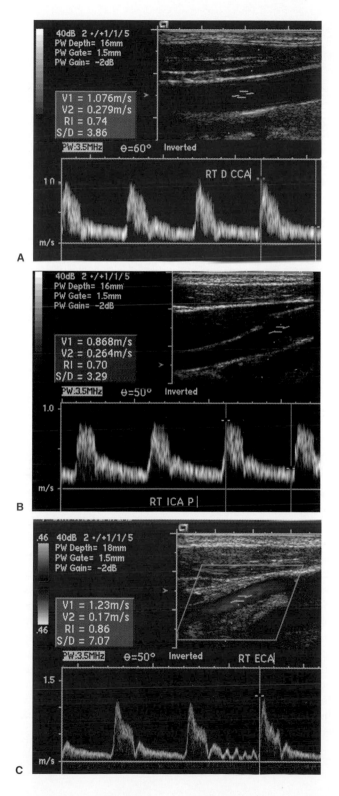

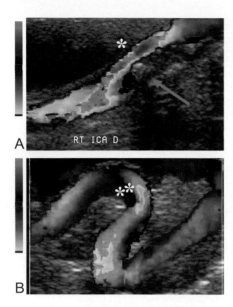

Figure 4.4 Color Doppler patterns. (A) Aliasing (*) at the site of an echolucent atherosclerotic plaque (arrow). (B) Reversal in flow (**) from the perspective of the color Doppler, as the vessel goes abruptly towards and away from the transducer. The red and blue regions in this instance are separated by a black line.

Diagnosis of stenosis

Abnormal flow patterns are evident at sites of arterial narrowing. Aliasing of the Doppler signal occurs when the velocities increase substantially at the site of stenosis. The maximal frequency shift exceeds one-half of the pulse repetition frequency (the Nyquist limit), and the frequency shifts cannot be processed properly. The color display becomes progressively lighter until it wraps around to display the lightest color signal of flow in the opposite direction (Figure 4.4A). In contrast, the color change with reverse flow demonstrates a black band (center band) between the red and blue flow (Figure 4.4B). The spectral Doppler display of aliasing displays the peak velocities below the baseline.

The spectral Doppler examination is used to quantify the stenosis[6,7], utilizing the peak systolic velocities, end-diastolic velocities, and ratios of the systolic velocities (Table 4.1). There are general values apparent across all criteria. An elevation in peak systolic velocity to greater than 125 cm s^{-1} is consistently seen when there is greater than 50% lumen narrowing. A peak systolic velocity greater than 230 cm s^{-1} generally identifies greater than 70% stenosis at the site of maximal stenosis (Figure 4.5). The peak systolic velocity is proportional to lumen narrowing for stenoses of 50–90%. There is turbulence and spectral broadening beyond the site of stenosis, with flow eddies contributing lower velocities in the flow profile. Flow reversal is evident just beyond the jet of a high-grade stenosis. An end-diastolic velocity greater than 100 cm s^{-1} also identifies high-grade stenosis, i.e. stenosis greater than 70–80%. There is a delay in upstroke in the spectral Doppler beyond the site of significant stenosis, termed a "tardus et parvus" waveform[8] (Figure 4.6).

Table 4.1 Velocity criteria for internal carotid artery stenosis.

Stenosis (%)	ICA PSV (cm s⁻¹)	Lumen narrowing	ICA EDV (cm s⁻¹)	ICA/CCA PSV
0	< 125	–	< 40	< 2
1–49	< 125	+	< 40	< 2
50–69	> 125	+	40–100	2–4
> 70	> 230	+	> 100	> 4
Subtotal occlusion	Widely variable	++	Widely variable	Widely variable
Total occlusion	0	–	0	0

CCA = common carotid artery; EDV = end-diastolic velocity; ICA = internal carotid artery; PSV = peak systolic velocity.

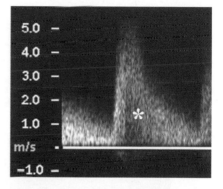

Figure 4.5 High-grade internal carotid artery stenosis. The peak systolic velocity is greater than 500 cm s⁻¹. The end-diastolic velocity is 150 cm s⁻¹. There is clear spectral broadening (*), consistent with the turbulence associated with the stenosis.

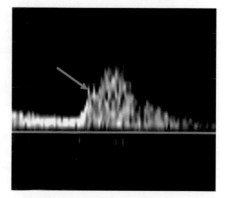

Figure 4.6 The "tardus et parvus" waveform with a delay in the upstroke indicated by the arrow. This is suggestive of a more proximal high-grade stenosis.

A stenosis of greater than 95% can cause the flow and the peak systolic velocity at the site of the stenosis to decrease. Low velocities coincident with a narrow lumen assessed by color Doppler or gray scale are referred to as the "string sign." This trickle of flow is consistent with subtotal occlusion. The lumen diameter at the stenosis can be compared with the contralateral arterial diameter to confirm that the narrow lumen and low flow are consistent with greater than

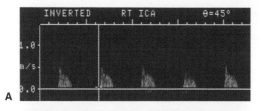

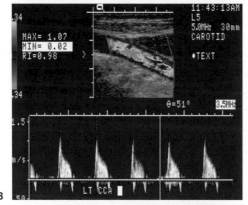

Figure 4.7 Evidence of carotid occlusion. (A) Low amplitude and the absence of diastolic flow are consistent with distal total occlusion of the vessel. Distal total occlusion is a high-resistance stake. (B) Absence of diastolic flow in the common carotid artery (CCA) waveform suggests that no CCA flow is reaching the low-resistance vascular bed of the brain. This finding suggests distal internal carotid artery (ICA) occlusion, and may also be found in brain death.

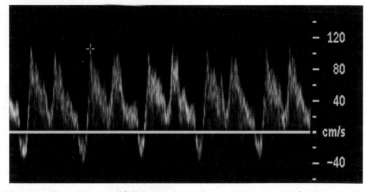

Figure 4.8 Internal carotid artery (ICA) spectral waveform in the presence of an intra-aortic balloon pump.

95% stenosis. Low velocities in the ICA with diminished diastolic flow are consistent with significant intracranial ICA stenosis (Figure 4.7A). The ratio of the ICA peak systolic velocity to the mid-CCA peak velocity is another means of identifying ICA stenosis. The ICA/CCA systolic velocity ratio can be used to further verify the degree of stenosis in patients with low cardiac output or severe aortic stenosis. A ratio greater than two is consistent with significant narrowing, while a ratio greater than four is consistent with high-grade stenosis. In the presence of an intra-aortic balloon pump, the first systolic peak is used to determine the velocity (Figure 4.8).

Similarly, low CCA velocities with absent diastolic flow suggest ipsilateral

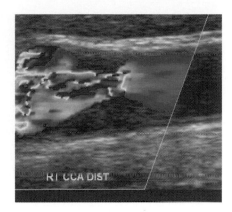

Figure 4.9 Common carotid artery (CCA) stenosis. Aliasing is evident at the site of lumen narrowing. The systolic velocity is 280 cm s⁻¹ at the site of stenosis and 00 cm s⁻¹ proximal to the stenosis. The distal to proximal ratio of four indicates greater than 75% stenosis.

ICA occlusion (Figure 4.7B). Waveforms with delayed upstroke and dampened velocities are consistent with stenosis proximal to the visualized CCA. Stenosis within the visualized portion of the CCA is rare (Figure 4.9). Such stenosis is graded by comparing the systolic velocity at the lesion to a more proximal systolic velocity. Doubling of the systolic velocity from proximal to distal indicates greater than 50% stenosis, and quadrupling of the velocity suggests greater than 75% stenosis. Tubular narrowing of the artery without a clear atherosclerosis plaque is consistent with arteritis or fibromuscular dysplasia.

Artifactual increase in systolic velocity

High-grade stenosis of the ECA can result in increased peak systolic velocities in the ipsilateral ICA. It is of paramount importance to distinguish ECA from ICA stenosis. Again, this can be performed by identifying ECA branches, or deflections in the ECA waveform secondary to tapping on the pre-auricular temporal artery. The outside curve of a tortuous vessel will have artifactually high systolic velocities. Systolic velocities are also disproportionately elevated on the side contralateral to a high-grade stenosis. Systemic conditions causing high cardiac output can also increase carotid velocities. Examples include hyperthyroidism or immediate post-exercise states.

Plaque evaluation

Atherosclerotic plaque is characterized by the amount, echogenicity, surface characteristics, and calcium content[9]. The amount of plaque is difficult to quantify. Transverse imaging and three-dimensional reconstruction may be useful in this regard. The use of harmonic imaging can also clarify plaque characteristics. The plaque density is characterized with respect to the surrounding tissue. Echolucent plaque is darker than surrounding tissue, while echodense plaque is hyperechoic with respect to the surrounding tissue (Figure 4.10). Echolucency can be secondary to high lipid concentration or hemorrhage within the plaque.

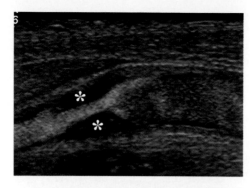

Figure 4.10 Echolucent atherosclerotic plaque (*) evident on both walls of the internal carotid artery (ICA). Contrast fills the lumen.

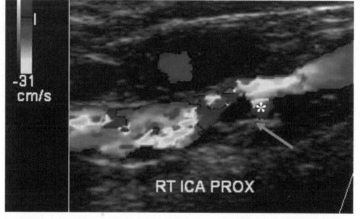

Figure 4.11 Plaque ulceration. The lumen is identified by color Doppler. The plaque (arrow) has mixed echogenicity, with an ulcer on the surface (*) identified by the blue color Doppler signal.

A high degree of echolucency is associated with an increased risk of cerebrovascular events[10]. The plaque surface is characterized as smooth, irregular, or ulcerated. Irregularity and ulceration suggest that a plaque is actively changing. Ulceration is identified by flow reversal within the ulcer pit (Figure 4.11), and is also a marker for increased stroke risk. Calcification within the plaque may identify sites of earlier plaque hemorrhage that have now healed. Extensively calcified plaque can result in a shadowing artifact and can limit ultrasound evaluation. The vessel must be examined from multiple angles in order to adequately assess the lumen.

Revascularization

The carotid anatomy is altered after endarterectomy[11]. The carotid bulb is absent, and patch material may be evident. Thrombus may be seen lining the

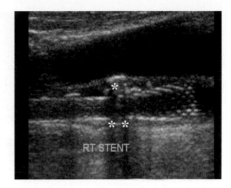

Figure 4.12 Carotid stent. The textured pattern of the carotid stent is most evident on the right. The plaque (*) has not been completely compressed by the stent. Shadowing artifact from calcium within the plaque is present (*).

lumen if the proximal ICA has been widened significantly. Intimal hyperplasia develops over months to years following endarterectomy. It appears as homogeneous, symmetric thickening of the arterial walls. Findings after carotid stenting are similar to those post-endarterectomy only in the loss of the carotid bulb. The carotid stent structure is evident on ultrasound (Figure 4.12). False elevation of peak systolic velocities is seen with the older, stiffer stent. It is essential to compare velocities over time in these cases. Another difference in the post-stent examination compared with the post-endarterectomy examination is the retention of atherosclerotic plaque post-stent. Calcified plaques can significantly distort the architecture of the stent. Post-revascularization (endarterectomy and stent) surveillance is important in order to detect restenosis and contralateral disease progression at yearly intervals.

Arterial wall evaluation

The arterial wall can also be evaluated for thickness, edema, and injury such as dissection. Ultrasound is used to evaluate the combined thickness of the intima plus the media[12]. This is most easily performed using the posterior wall of the distal CCA. The measurement is made from the intima lumen interface to the media adventitia border (Figure 4.13A). The thickness is normally less than 0.6 mm in a young, healthy population. Further thickening is thought to represent the early stages of atherosclerosis, and is associated with increased cardiovascular risk. The small value of the measurements makes it difficult to utilize this technique for serial evaluations in an individual. The arterial wall is also diffusely thickened in arteritis (Figure 4.13B). The inflammation results in predominantly echolucent thickening of the media and adventitia. The degree and echolucency of the wall have been used to gauge the degree of active inflammation in vessels with arteritis. A final abnormality in the arterial wall is trauma and dissection (Figure 4.13C). The dissection flap can be difficult to appreciate and requires careful gray scale evaluation. The abnormal flow patterns created with ICA dissection can result in marked variation in the ICA waveform.

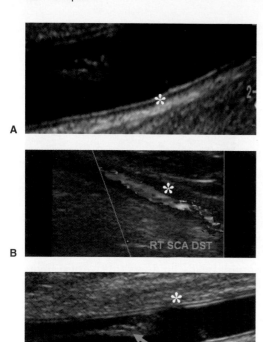

A

B

C

Figure 4.13 Carotid wall evaluation.
(A) The intima media thickness can be
evaluated by measuring the combined
thickness (*) of the intima (white line) and
media (black line). The second white line is
the adventitia. This is not included in the
measurement. (B) Giant cell arteritis. The
wall of the vessel is diffusely thickened and
hypoechoic. (C) Trauma to the carotid
artery. A disruption of the wall (*) is evident
at the site of inadvertent cannulation.
Thrombus is seen extending into the lumen
distal to the puncture site (arrow).

Pulsatile masses

Pulsatile neck masses are most often caused by tortuosity of the carotid arteries
(Figure 4.4). Trauma to the carotid arteries can result in aneurysm formation.
Aneurysm is defined as a doubling in arterial diameter. Aneurysms are extremely rare in the absence of trauma. They may occur in concert with other
aneurysmal disease. Evaluations of aneurysm must include careful assessment
for the presence or absence of thrombus. Soft tissue masses can displace the
carotid arteries and create the impression of a pulsatile mass. Enlarged lymph
nodes are the most common cause of this phenomenon, while carotid body
tumor is rarer. Carotid body tumor is identified by its location at the bifurcation
and results in splaying of the ICA and ECA course. The marked vascularity of
this tumor is evident on color Doppler examination.

Vertebral artery evaluation

The vertebral artery is evaluated with the probe in a longitudinal position and
beginning with a clear color Doppler duplex image of the CCA. The probe is then
directed posteriorly and laterally. The vertebral artery will be intermittently
seen between the shadows of the vertebral spinous processes (Figure 4.14).
The vertebral vein will be anterior to the artery and will normally demonstrate
flow away from the head. Pulsed wave Doppler evaluation is performed with

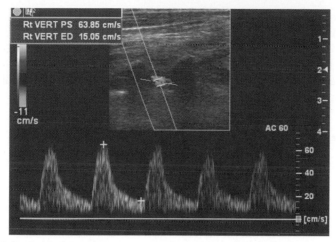

Figure 4.14 Duplex of the vertebral artery. The red color flow signal identifies the vertebral artery as it passes through the spinous processes. The spectral waveform has a low-resistance pattern, with continuous flow during diastole.

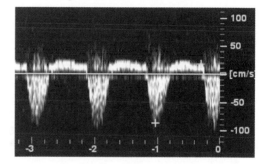

Figure 4.15 Reversal of vertebral artery flow.

the sample cursor aligned parallel to the inner wall and at a 60° angle to the insonation beam. The evaluation of vertebral artery hemodynamics relies on careful assessment of the waveform characteristics[13]. A low-resistance spectral waveform is typical of the vertebral artery (Figure 4.14). The absence of diastolic flow suggests distal total occlusion of the distal vertebral artery. Retrograde, high-resistance flow in the vertebral artery suggests ipsilateral subclavian stenosis; subclavian steal may be present. Vertebral artery stenosis is difficult to define, as spectral Doppler cannot continuously march through the vessel. Peak systolic velocities greater than 125 cm s^{-1} are suggestive of significant stenosis. If the vertebral artery waveform is bifid or biphasic, a presteal phenomenon is possible. The artery can be re-evaluated after inflating and deflating a blood pressure cuff on the ipsilateral arm. The vertebral artery flow will be reversed on subsequent scanning in the presence of subclavian steal (Figure 4.15). The proximal subclavian artery is then evaluated for evidence of discrete increases in velocity to greater than 125 cm s^{-1}, consistent with stenosis, and for the presence of post-stenotic waveforms.

Cervical carotid artery examination requires careful and methodical assessment of the carotid, vertebral, and subclavian arteries. Gray scale, color Doppler, and spectral Doppler waveform analysis all have integral roles in this evaluation.

Reference list

1 Manzi S, Selzer F, Sutton-Tyrrell K, *et al.* Prevalence and risk factors of carotid plaque in women with systemic lupus erythematosus. Arthritis Rheum 1999; 42:51–60.

2 Ebrahim S, Papacosta O, Whincup P, *et al.* Carotid plaque, intima media thickness, cardiovascular risk factors, and prevalent cardiovascular disease in men and women: the British Regional Heart Study. Stroke 1999; 30:841–850.

3 Salonen JT, Salonen R. Arterial wall thickness, carotid atherosclerosis and the risk of myocardial infarction and cerebrovascular stroke. In: Touboul P, Crouse III JC (eds), Intima-Media Thickness and Atherosclerosis: Predicting the Risk, pp. 97–104. New York, NY: Parthenon Publishing Group, 1997.

4 O'Leary DH, Polak JF, Kronmal RA, *et al.* Distribution and correlates of sonographically detected carotid artery disease in the Cardiovascular Health Study. The CHS Collaborative Research Group. Stroke 1992; 23:1752–1760.

5 O'Leary DI I, Polak JF, Kronmal RA, Manolio TA, Burke GL, Wolfson SK Jr. Carotid-artery intima and media thickness as a risk factor for myocardial infarction and stroke in older adults. Cardiovascular Health Study Collaborative Research Group [comment]. N Engl J Med 1999; 340:14–22.

6 AbuRahma AF, Robinson PA, Strickler DL, Alberts S, Young L. Proposed new duplex classification for threshold stenoses used in various symptomatic and asymptomatic carotid endarterectomy trials. Ann Vasc Surg 1998; 12:349–358.

7 Grant EG, Benson CB, Moneta GL, *et al.* Carotid artery stenosis: gray-scale and Doppler US diagnosis—Society of Radiologists in Ultrasound Consensus Conference. Radiology 2003; 229:340–346.

8 Kotval PS. Doppler waveform parvus and tardus. A sign of proximal flow obstruction. J Ultrasound Med 1989; 8:435–440.

9 Joakimsen O, Bonaa KH, Stensland-Bugge E. Reproducibility of ultrasound assessment of carotid plaque occurrence, thickness, and morphology. The Tromso Study. Stroke 1997; 28:2201–2207.

10 Takiuchi S, Rakugi H, Honda K, *et al.* Quantitative ultrasonic tissue characterization can identify high-risk atherosclerotic alteration in human carotid arteries. Circulation 2000; 102:766–770.

11 Baker WH, Koustas G, Burke K, Littooy FN, Greisler HP. Intraoperative duplex scanning and late carotid artery stenosis. J Vasc Surg 1994; 19:829–832; discussion 832–833.

12 Persson J, Formgren J, Israelsson B, Berglund G. Ultrasound-determined intima-media thickness and atherosclerosis. Direct and indirect validation. Arteriosclerosis Thrombosis 1994; 14:261–264.

13 Rohren EM, Kliewer MA, Carroll BA, Hertzberg BS. A spectrum of Doppler waveforms in the carotid and vertebral arteries. Am J Roentgenol 2003; 181:1695–1704.

PART III

 Aorta

5 Thoracic Aorta Imaging

Paul A. Tunick and Itzhak Kronzon

This chapter concentrates on several aortic syndromes. Although they may cause separate clinical pictures, they may also be associated with each other in the same patient. The aortic syndromes discussed include aortic atherosclerosis, aortic dissection, aortic intramural hematoma, and aortic aneurysm.

Diagnostic tests

Transthoracic echocardiography (TTE) may occasionally demonstrate large aortic arch plaque in patients with stroke or other embolic phenomena, intimal flaps in patients with dissection, intramural hematomas, and aortic aneurysms. However, the sensitivity of TTE is limited, as is its resolution. This low resolution makes it difficult to measure the most important prognostic factor in stroke patients—plaque thickness. The low resolution of TTE also makes it easier to miss mobile thrombi, intramural hematomas, and dissection flaps. Although the TTE window allows for the visualization of the ascending aorta, the more distal aorta is less accurately imaged.

The aorta may be evaluated by other imaging technologies, including magnetic resonance imaging (MRI), computed tomography (CT), and contrast aortography. The sensitivity of these tests is comparable with that of transesophageal echocardiography (TEE). Each of these techniques has its own benefits and limitations. One major limitation of MRI, CT, and angiography is the need to transport the patient to the radiology suite for imaging, thus interfering with the critical care of the patient and with prompt diagnosis.

Currently, TEE is the diagnostic test of choice in patients with stroke or other embolic phenomena, and is also a rapidly available modality for the diagnosis of dissection, intramural hematoma, and aneurysm. In these latter conditions, when early diagnosis may be life-saving, TEE is also the diagnostic imaging procedure of choice.

Transesophageal echocardiography technique

TEE is relatively noninvasive, has advantages over MRI for the diagnosis of severe aortic plaque, and has a low complication rate. Although conscious sedation may be used, and is recommended in patients who may have aortic dissection and have no contraindication, the procedure is often performed in the awake patient. A complete evaluation of the thoracic aorta may be finished in approximately 5 min, and there is complete visualization, except for a small part of the ascending aorta which is masked by the tracheal air column. The aortic arch and descending thoracic aorta, critical in patients with thromboemboli or atheroemboli, may be fully examined.

The patient is given local anesthesia (e.g. Cetacaine spray). Care should be taken to anesthetize the oropharynx rather than just the tongue or palate. Excessive anesthetic doses should be avoided to prevent paralysis of the swallowing mechanism or neurologic toxicity. Methemoglobinemia is an unusual complication, and may be recognized by monitoring oxygenation saturation (with a pulse oximeter). Electrocardiographic and noninvasive blood pressure monitoring is also routine, and is especially necessary if conscious sedation is employed. Because of the local anesthesia, patients must not eat or drink for 90 min. If no sedation is used, there is no post-procedure care necessary, and patients may resume their activities (except for oral intake) immediately. After conscious sedation, a 2 h monitoring period is prudent, and outpatients should be accompanied home without driving. The presence of esophageal pathology is the only relative or absolute contraindication to the TEE procedure (depending on the severity of the esophageal lesion). Zenker's diverticulum may be recognized when there is resistance to passage of the probe past the upper esophagus. To avoid esophageal damage, it is imperative that the probe be advanced gently, and not be advanced further if there is resistance. TEE may be safely performed on unconscious, intubated patients in the intensive care unit (ICU) or operating room, with special care not to advance the probe against resistance, as the patient will not be able to report discomfort. In smaller patients (e.g. ≤ 100 lb), a pediatric probe is available, with only a small loss of resolution.

The thoracic aorta is examined in two stages. First, the aortic valve, sinuses of Valsalva, proximal coronary arteries, and ascending aorta are visualized, using multiple transducer angles between 0° and 120°. The left ventricular outflow tract, aortic valve, and ascending aorta are especially well seen with a transducer angle of 120°. The second part of the examination involves visualization of the descending aorta and aortic arch.

With the transducer pointing anteriorly and scanning at 0°, the probe is advanced to the level of the aortic valve. With slight withdrawal and anteflexion of the probe tip, the sinuses of Valsalva and the coronary arteries are visualized. Frequently, it is possible to visualize the ostium of the left coronary artery. The left main coronary artery can be detected at the level of the left atrial appendage, and can be followed to its bifurcation into the left anterior descending and circumflex artery. Visualization of the ostium of the right coronary artery is more difficult because of its anterior location. However, with either anteflexion or retroflexion of the tip of the probe, clear images of the proximal right coronary artery may be seen. Ostial or proximal coronary artery stenosis may be diagnosed using color and pulsed wave Doppler. Whilst withdrawing the probe, it is possible to see serial views of the proximal ascending aorta at 0°.

The ascending aorta can then be further imaged by advancing the probe slightly and changing the transducer angle to 90–120°. Images of the upper ascending aorta and proximal aortic arch can be obtained by slight anteflexion and withdrawal of the probe.

The second half of the TEE examination of the thoracic aorta involves the imaging of the descending thoracic aorta and the entire aortic arch. The examination begins at the level of the stomach, with the transducer at 0°. From the images of the heart obtained as described above, the probe is rotated counterclockwise until the characteristic round cross-section of the descending aorta is seen. Occasionally, the upper abdominal aorta, superior mesenteric and celiac arteries may be visualized. Serial tomographic slices of the aorta can be obtained by withdrawing the probe. A continuous clockwise rotation is necessary to keep the aorta in view whilst the probe is withdrawn as a result of the changing relationship between the aorta and the esophagus. At the level of the stomach, the transducer is pointed posteriorly as, at this level, the aorta lies posterior to the stomach. By mid-thorax, the aorta lies just to the left of the esophagus; at the level of the aortic arch, the esophagus has become posterior to the aorta. Eventually, the aortic arch will appear in the left-hand portion of the screen whilst imaging at 0°. With clockwise rotation, the entire arch and distal ascending aorta may be visualized, with the ascending aorta appearing furthest from the transducer.

Long-axis views of the descending aorta can easily be obtained at various levels by rotating the transducer angle to 90° as the probe is being withdrawn from the stomach to the views of the arch. Similarly, while the aortic arch is seen at 0°, rotating the transducer angle to 90° will reveal excellent images of the aortic arch in cross-section, as well as proximal views of the carotid and subclavian arteries.

Doppler echocardiography is an important adjunct in the evaluation of patients with aortic dissection and intramural hematoma. In dissection, color flow Doppler imaging demonstrates the blood flow pattern in the true and false lumens, and the communications between the two. Color flow imaging is also important for the diagnosis of intramural hematoma, in which there is no flow within the wall/hematoma (only in the aortic lumen).

Aortic atherosclerosis

Arterio-arterial embolism originating from an atherosclerotic plaque in the thoracic aorta (Figure 5.1) may lead to the occlusion of distal arterial branches, with resultant organ infarction caused by either of two mechanisms: small- to medium-sized artery occlusion as a result of atheroembolism, or medium to large artery occlusion as a result of thromboembolism. The first has been recognized for many years as the syndrome of cholesterol crystal embolization, or the "blue toe syndrome," which usually comprises one or more of the following — renal failure, blue toes, livedo reticularis, and intestinal infarction[1]. The second phenomenon, thromboembolism originating from an atherosclerotic plaque in the thoracic aorta, has been more recently recognized as being much more frequent than classic atheroembolism syndrome, with organ damage caused by

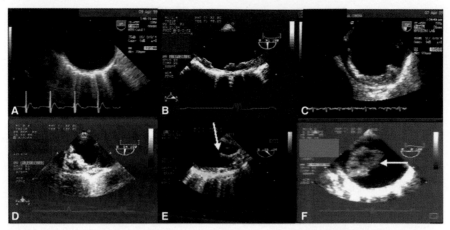

Figure 5.1 Thoracic aortic atherosclerosis. A. Transesophageal echocardiography (TEE): normal descending aorta, no intimal plaque (0°). B. TEE: severe (5 mm) descending aorta plaque (91°) with severe ulceration. C. TEE: very severe (7 mm) aortic arch plaque (72°). D. TEE: very severe (10 mm) aortic arch plaque (74°) which occupies nearly half of the aortic lumen. E. TEE: severe descending aorta plaque with long mobile thrombus (arrow). F. TEE: severe distal aortic arch plaque with huge mobile thrombus (arrow).

thrombus embolization from unstable plaques in the thoracic aorta[2]. This thromboembolism from aortic plaque is a major cause of stroke or transient ischemic attack (TIA), similar in prevalence to carotid artery disease and atrial fibrillation in patients with stroke. Thromboembolism from unstable aortic plaque may also cause limb ischemia or damage to the kidneys or intestine.

The traditional atherosclerosis risk factors of male sex, hypertension, age, and smoking have been positively correlated with severe thoracic aortic atherosclerotic plaque seen on TEE in a population-based study[3]. Amongst those with plaque, the odds of complex atherosclerosis (defined as plaque ≥ 4 mm measured on TEE, ulceration, and/or superimposed mobile thrombi) increased as the ambulatory systolic blood pressure increased (odds ratio of 1.43 for each 10 mmHg increase; 95% confidence interval, 1.10–1.87). Complex aortic plaque was also correlated with hypertension treatment, controlling for age and history of smoking.

Other risk factors for atherosclerosis have more recently come to light, especially homocysteine levels, which are correlated not only with clinical atherosclerosis[4], but also with the degree of plaque burden in the thoracic aorta on TEE[5]. It is thought that endothelial damage by homocysteine may cause plaque development.

Current theories also point to inflammation in the pathogenesis of atherosclerosis and the syndromes or atheroembolism and thromboembolism[6]. There is great interest in the levels of inflammation markers, such as the highly sensitive C-reactive protein (CRP). Much evidence points to the fact that CRP levels are a risk factor for atherosclerosis and its complications[7]; there is also some evidence that rather than just being a marker for inflammation, CRP could itself be etiologic. CRP levels have been found to be associated with plaque severity in the thoracic aorta.

Atheroembolism

Atheroembolism is an uncommon but lethal syndrome. Patients with atheroembolism have a diffuse showering of the distal arteries with cholesterol crystals originating from arterial plaque (usually in the aorta; the syndrome may also involve the iliac, carotid, and coronary arteries)[8]. These crystals lodge in small- and medium-sized vessels, producing damage to vital organs. When this occurs in the lower extremities, it is often called "blue toe syndrome," and the syndrome also commonly affects the kidneys. The upper extremities and the intestine are less often affected.

Atheroembolism syndrome was found in only 1% of 519 patients with severe thoracic aortic plaque on TEE during a follow-up time of more than 3 years[9]. Similarly, in the Stroke Prevention in Atrial Fibrillation (SPAF)-III trial, it occurred in only one of 134 warfarin-treated patients with severe aortic plaque[10].

The presenting symptoms of atheroembolism syndrome are often nonspecific, and this may lead to confusion with other systemic illnesses. The differential diagnosis is large, and includes thrombotic arterial occlusion, vasospastic disorders (Raynaud's phenomenon or chronic pernio), cyanotic congenital heart disease, secondary syphilis, and pheochromocytoma[11]. Atheroembolism syndrome may also be mistaken for syphilis, endocarditis, Whipple disease, tuberculosis, arteritis, aortic dissection, atrial myxoma, lymphoma, and renal cell carcinoma. In addition to blue toes, skin findings may include ulceration and livedo reticularis (a reticulated erythema of the skin which is blanchable).

Atheroembolism may also cause acute renal failure, a life-threatening manifestation. Characteristic cholesterol clefts on biopsy were found in 7% of 259 patients of > 60 years of age with acute renal failure[12]. Renal failure most often occurs after invasive vascular procedures, although it may also occur spontaneously. The course of renal failure may be steadily downhill (resulting in the need for dialysis), relatively benign, or there may be a stuttering course with additional showers of cholesterol crystals. Although renal insufficiency following invasive vascular procedures, such as angiography, is usually blamed on toxicity from the contrast used, atheroembolism should always be considered in elderly patients or in those who have other manifestations of atherosclerosis.

In addition to skin and renal findings, gastrointestinal bleeding may be present, as well as cholesterol crystals in the retina (Hollenhorst plaques). The intestine, pancreas, liver, and gallbladder may also be rarely affected by atheroembolism.

Atheroembolism syndrome may be spontaneous in approximately one-half of patients, and is precipitated by angiography or surgery in the other half. Rarely, atheroemboli may be precipitated by trauma. There are reports of atheroembolism occurring after treatment with the anticoagulants warfarin and heparin[13–15], and these drugs are often thought to be etiologic (with plaque hemorrhage as the precipitating factor). However, as noted above, the syndrome occurs very uncommonly in patients treated with anticoagulants. In a study of 519 patients treated for severe aortic plaque[9], it occurred in only two patients on warfarin.

The diagnosis of atheroembolism requires a high index of suspicion. If renal failure, abdominal pain, or blue toes and livedo reticularis occur following cardiac catheterization, angiography, vascular surgery, or blunt trauma to the abdomen, the syndrome should be at the top of the list of possibilities. This is especially true in a patient with an abdominal aortic aneurysm, or in the so-called "vasculopathic" patient.

Laboratory testing may reveal elevations in the white blood cell count, or in the blood urea nitrogen and creatinine. There may also be abnormalities on urinalysis (sometimes with eosinophiluria), and peripheral eosinophilia may also be present.

The definitive diagnosis of atheroembolism comes from biopsy, surgical pathology, or autopsy. However, less invasive testing may be suggestive of the diagnosis. The presence of Hollenhorst plaques, aneurysmal disease on diagnostic ultrasound or other imaging, or severe thoracic aortic plaque on TEE may lead to the correct diagnosis. Recently, mobile small particles in transit from severe aortic plaque were observed on TEE in a patient who later died after multisystem involvement from atheroemboli[16].

Thromboembolism originating from thoracic aortic plaque

Thromboembolism originates from unstable atherosclerotic plaques, which, when they rupture, are the sites of clot formation. There is resultant organ damage when thrombi detach from the plaques, travel downstream, and lodge in medium-sized or large arteries. Severe thoracic aortic plaque as an embolic source has been recognized on TEE since 1990[2]. The prevalence of severe thoracic aortic plaque, seen on TEE in stroke patients (21–27%), is of the same order of magnitude as the prevalence of carotid artery disease (10–13%) and atrial fibrillation (18–30%) reported in two large series of consecutive stroke patients[17,18].

Thromboembolism from atherosclerotic plaques in the thoracic aorta is responsible for a significant number of strokes that were formerly called "cryptogenic," in the same way as carotid artery disease became recognized as the etiology of many "cryptogenic" strokes when the significance of carotid atherosclerosis was reported by C. Miller Fisher in the 1950s.

The risk of stroke in patients with severe thoracic aortic plaque is high: strokes occur in 12% of patients in 1 year[19,20], and peripheral emboli in an additional 20% of patients[19]. In a study of 519 patients with severe thoracic aortic plaque on TEE, who were followed for an average of 3 years[9], there were 111 embolic events (21%). There were 56 strokes, 39 TIAs, and 16 peripheral emboli. Thromboembolism from thoracic aortic plaque may damage multiple organs in the same patient. For example, leg ischemia may occur together with stroke, intestinal embolization, or renal infarction.

One particularly severe complication of thoracic aortic plaque is stroke, which occurs during heart surgery employing cardiopulmonary bypass. Although intra-operative stroke is often blamed on the bypass pump, or air embolism, it is often caused by cannulation of the aorta for the institution of cardiopulmonary bypass in patients with severe aortic arch plaque. Strokes occurred in 12% of 268 patients with severe thoracic plaque on TEE[21] —this is six times the average stroke risk during heart surgery employing cardiopulmonary bypass. These strokes are especially severe, with a hospital mortality of 39%. More subtle forms of cerebral damage ("cognitive dysfunction") could also be due to embolization from thoracic aortic plaque.

Although thromboembolism may be precipitated by instrumentation, it frequently occurs spontaneously when unstable plaques undergo plaque rupture and subsequent thrombosis. TEE shows that the resulting thrombi are mobile, and such mobile thrombi were detected in 127 of 519 patients (24%) with severe thoracic aortic plaque[9].

The most important measurable characteristic of aortic plaque is the plaque thickness as seen on TEE. The French Aortic Plaque and Stroke Group found that the odds ratio for stroke in patients with plaques of < 1 mm in thickness was 1.0 (no increased risk). For plaques measuring 1.0–3.9 mm, the odds ratio was 3.9, and for plaques of ≥ 4 mm in thickness it was much higher, 13.8[17]. The French study also lends support to the etiologic role of aortic arch plaque in stroke, as the odds ratio for stroke in patients with severe plaques in the descending aorta (which would not embolize to the brain) was only 1.5 vs. 13.8 for patients with severe plaques in the arch.

Although some of the mobile lesions superimposed on atherosclerotic plaques may be part of the plaque itself ("debris"), early case reports of two patients who underwent aortic arch surgery documented that these mobile components were in fact thrombi, which were removed from the aortic plaque itself, as well as from the femoral artery and subclavian artery, after embolization[22,23]. This has been corroborated pathologically in additional patients, including an autopsy study which documented aortic thrombi in 17 of 120 consecutive autopsies, as well as a significant association of complex plaque (thrombi, ulceration) with prior emboli[24].

The critical prognostic importance of plaque thickness has been stressed above. When the largest plaque has been visually identified, the image should be frozen for measurement. Intimal plaque thickness is measured from the largest luminal protrusion up to, but not including, the adventitia. Superimposed mobile thrombi, as well as ulceration or calcification, should be noted. Whereas thrombi and ulceration are high-risk characteristics, plaque calcification has been found (by the French Aortic Plaque and Stroke Group) to be present when the risk of stroke is lower. Calcified plaques may represent more stable lesions, less likely to undergo plaque rupture, thrombosis, and subsequent embolization.

Aortic dissection

Aortic dissection is a medical emergency. Unfortunately, the pain associated with dissection is frequently atypical. Its axial nature may lead to confusion of dissection with other causes of head, neck, chest, back, abdominal, or leg pain. If dissection goes undiagnosed, there may be a high risk, with acute mortality rates of 1–2% per hour.

As noted above, TEE is the diagnostic procedure of choice[25,26]. It can make the diagnosis of dissection at the bedside, and can easily be performed on critically ill patients without the need for contrast or ionizing radiation. The hallmark of the diagnosis of dissection is the demonstration of an intimal flap (Figure 5.2). It is critical to define the most proximal extent of the dissection, as those dissections involving the ascending aorta (Type A) are an immediate surgical indication because of the high acute mortality rates in unoperated patients. Dissections that

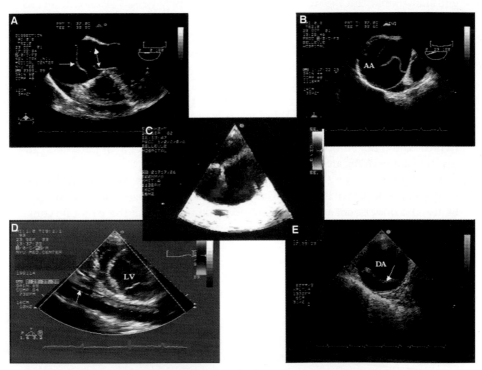

Figure 5.2 Aortic dissection. A. Transesophageal echocardiography (TEE): ascending aortic dissection. Note the intimal flap (arrow) 1–2 cm distal to the aortic valve (double-headed arrow). B. TEE: ascending aortic dissection. Note the two pieces of intimal flap, which were mobile. C. TEE: descending aortic dissection, color Doppler. The communication between the lumens through a hole in the intimal flap is demonstrated by blue flow on color Doppler. D. TTE: descending aortic dissection. Note the intimal flap (arrow). Flow (as seen on color Doppler in red) is limited to the true lumen. E. TEE: descending aortic dissection. Note the intimal flap (arrow) in the descending aorta (DA). In this case, the smaller true lumen is compressed by the larger false lumen.

do not involve the ascending aorta (Type B) may be managed medically if they are uncomplicated by expansion, bleeding, compression of vital structures, or compromised flow to vital organs. These complications of dissection may also be diagnosed by ultrasound examination/echocardiography.

The complications of Type A dissection include aortic rupture with exsanguination or pericardial tamponade, myocardial infarction (as a result of interference with coronary flow), stroke, and acute aortic regurgitation with pulmonary edema. All of these complications may be diagnosed using TEE, and they should be aggressively ruled out during the TEE examination. A special attempt should be made to identify the origins of the coronary arteries, the aortic arch vessels, the major abdominal arteries (celiac axis, superior mesenteric artery, and renal arteries), and the lower extremity vessels. Vessels below the diaphragm should be evaluated using abdominal ultrasonography at the time of TEE. Compromised blood flow may be a result of occlusion by the dissection flap or because the vessels may arise from an underperfused false lumen. In the case of the latter, the intimal flap may be fenestrated by a balloon using TEE guidance, thereby improving blood flow to compromised beds[27].

The intimal flap of the aortic dissection may be easily recognized on TEE as a linear echodensity that is within the aortic lumen (Figure 5.2). The mobility of the flap may depend on the acuity of the dissection, as clot formation in the false lumen may reduce or stop flap mobility. Rarely, when the intimal tear is circumferential, a sleeve-like flap may prolapse through the aortic valve in diastole[28].

Color Doppler should be used to demonstrate flow within the true and false lumens, and also to look for the communication(s) between the two. The separation of flow between true and false lumens is characteristic of dissection (Figure 5.2) and may be helpful in the differentiation of true dissection flaps from linear artifacts within the aorta (which do not divide the blood flow). Aortic regurgitation may be the result of dilation of the aortic ring, disruption of the architecture, and support of the aortic leaflets by the dissection, or of a prolapsing intimal sleeve (see above).

Echocardiography is useful in the follow-up of aortic dissection. It can evaluate surgical results, with visualization of intra-aortic conduits (grafts) and, in some cases, the native aortic "wrap" which is sometimes left around an ascending aortic conduit. With time, the space between the conduit and the "wrap" thromboses and blood flow is limited to the conduit lumen unless there is a partial dehiscence. The function of the aortic valve (which may be a native valve in its original or re-implanted position, or a prosthesis alone or in combination with a composite graft) should be evaluated. In those patients who are followed medically, echocardiography can demonstrate characteristic changes. Frequently with time, the flap becomes less mobile, the flow between the two lumens decreases, and the false lumen thromboses.

Aortic intramural hematoma

In intramural hematoma (Figure 5.3), there is bleeding within the wall of the

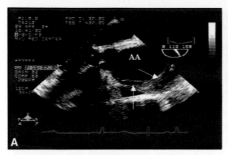 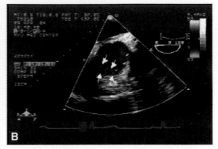

Figure 5.3 Aortic intramural hematoma. A: transesophageal echocardiography (TEE), 110°, of an ascending aortic intramural hematoma ("noncommunicating dissection"). There is a thickening of the anterior aortic wall, representing a hematoma within the wall of the ascending aorta (AA) (the arrows point to the intimal and the adventitial surfaces of the hematoma). The intimal surface (top arrow) is smooth. B: TEE, 0°, with color Doppler, of an ascending aortic intramural hematoma. The arrows outline the intramural hematoma, which appears as a thickened wall. It is distinguished from a plaque by the smooth intimal surface. Color flow Doppler demonstrates that flow is limited to the aortic lumen, and does not enter the hematoma.

aorta and a hematoma is contained between the layers of the wall. The intima is intact, without a tear, and thus there is no communication between the blood within the wall and the aortic lumen. Therefore, there are no false and true lumens; intramural hematoma has been referred to as a "noncommunicating dissection." There are two possible mechanisms for the development of intramural hematoma: bleeding from the vasa vasorum and penetrating atherosclerotic ulcer. This entity has similar predisposing factors to dissection. Both conditions are more common in hypertensive patients, cystic medial necrosis, and trauma (spontaneous and iatrogenic). An intramural hematoma may be found in 15% of patients studied for a suspected dissection, and it has the same presenting symptoms as dissection. As in dissection, TEE is the diagnostic procedure of choice[29].

The characteristic TEE findings (Figure 5.3) are uniform thickening (≥ 7 mm) of the aortic wall, sometimes containing heterogeneous areas caused by blood in different stages of clotting. Color Doppler should always be performed to ensure that there is no false lumen (no blood flow within the wall). The external aortic diameter is frequently increased, and intimal plaque and calcification are displaced towards the aortic lumen.

Approximately one-third of intramural hematomas will rupture into the mediastinum, pleura, pericardium, or abdomen, an additional third will progress to a typical communicating dissection, and the final third will resolve spontaneously. Because of the high complication rate when the ascending aorta is involved, immediate surgery is indicated. As in typical dissection, if the descending aorta is the area involved, the patient may be followed medically unless there are complications (bleeding, rupture, compression of vital structures, or branch artery occlusion). Monitoring of the patient with repeat imaging is indicated to detect an increase in size or other complication. It is possible

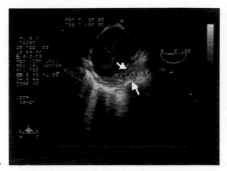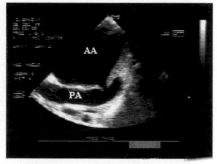

A   B

Figure 5.4 Aortic aneurysm. A: transesophageal echocardiography (TEE) of a large (6.5 cm) descending aortic aneurysm. Note the irregular mural thrombus (arrows) seen from approximately 3 o'clock to 7 o'clock. There are swirling echoes ("smoke") of spontaneous echo contrast within the lumen of the aneurysm, indicating stasis. B: intra-operative epiaortic echo of an ascending aortic (AA) aneurysm with rupture into the main pulmonary artery (PA).

that intramural hematoma and dissection are different stages of the same condition[30].

Aortic aneurysm

Aortic aneurysms (Figure 5.4) may be visualized in any part of the thoracic aorta. They may be saccular or fusiform, and may be associated with other aortic pathology, such as atheroma or dissection. Aneurysms are most commonly seen in patients with hypertensive and atherosclerotic disease, but are also a hallmark of hereditary abnormalities of connective tissue (such as Marfan's syndrome) and of various inflammatory and infectious conditions (such as Takayasu's and giant cell arteritis and syphilis).

Thoracic aneurysms are frequently asymptomatic. However, they may present with pain or compression syndromes (e.g. superior vena cava syndrome and Horner's syndrome). Aneurysmal deformation of the aortic root may result in aortic valvular regurgitation. Stagnation of blood within the aneurysm is common; spontaneous echo contrast ("smoke") is frequently visualized (Figure 5.4). Thrombus formation within the lumen of the aortic aneurysm (Figure 5.4) is not uncommon, and distal embolization may cause stroke or peripheral organ damage.

The most dangerous complication is rupture. The aneurysm may rupture into an adjacent cardiac chamber (as in rupture of a sinus of Valsalva aneurysm) or into another blood vessel (as shown in Figure 5.4, where an ascending thoracic aneurysm has ruptured into the pulmonary artery). Rupture into the pericardium will result in tamponade, and rupture into the pleural space may lead to exsanguination.

Accurate determination of the thoracic aneurysm diameter is crucial in making therapeutic, surgical, or interventional decisions, and precise measurement is possible using TEE, MRI, or CT scanning. TEE may also be valuable for intra-operative monitoring and in the post-operative evaluation of surgical repair or stent placement.

Reference list

1 Fine MJ, Kapoor W, Falanga V. Cholesterol crystal embolization: a review of 221 cases in the English literature. Angiology 1987; 38:769–784.

2 Tunick PA, Kronzon I. Protruding atherosclerotic plaque in the aortic arch of patients with systemic embolization: a new finding seen by transesophageal echocardiography. Am Heart J 1990; 120:658–660.

3 Agmon Y, Khandheria BK, Meissner I, et al. Independent association of high blood pressure and aortic atherosclerosis: a population-based study. Circulation 2000; 102:2087–2093.

4 von Eckardstein A, Malinow MR, Upson B, et al. Effects of age, lipoproteins, and hemostatic parameters on the role of homocyst(e)inemia as a cardiovascular risk factor in men. Arterioscler Thromb 1994; 14:460–464.

5 Konecky N, Malinow MR, Tunick PA, et al. Correlation between plasma homocyst(e)ine and aortic atherosclerosis. Am Heart J 1997; 133:534–540.

6 Fan J, Watanabe T. Inflammatory reactions in the pathogenesis of atherosclerosis. J Atheroscler Thromb 2003; 10:63–71.

7 Blake GJ, Ridker PM. C-reactive protein and other inflammatory risk markers in acute coronary syndromes. J Am Coll Cardiol 2003; 41:S37–S42.

8 Olin JW. Other peripheral arterial diseases. In: Goldman C (ed.), Textbook of Medicine, 21st edn., p. 362. Philadelphia: W. B. Saunders, 2000.

9 Tunick PA, Nayar AC, Goodkin GM, et al. for the NYU Atheroma Group. Effect of treatment on the incidence of stroke and other emboli in 519 patients with severe thoracic aortic plaque. Am J Cardiol 2002; 90:1320–1325.

10 The Stroke Prevention in Atrial Fibrillation Investigators Committee on Echocardiography. Transesophageal echocardiography correlates of thromboembolism in high-risk patients with nonvalvular atrial fibrillation. Ann Intern Med 1998; 128:639–647.

11 Abdelmalek MF, Spittell PC. 79-year-old woman with blue toes. Mayo Clin Proc 1995; 70:292–295.

12 Haas M, Spargo BH, Wit EJ, Meehan SM. Etiologies and outcome of acute renal insufficiency in older adults: a renal biopsy study of 259 cases. Am J Kidney Dis 2000; 35:433–447.

13 Ribera Pibernat M, Bigata Viscasillas X, Fuentes Gonzalez MJ, et al. [Cholesterol embolism disease: study of 16 cases]. Rev Clin Esp 2000; 200:659–663.

14 Nevelsteen A, Kutten M, Lacroix H, Suy R. Oral anticoagulant therapy: a precipitating factor in the pathogenesis of cholesterol embolization. Acta Chir Belg 1992; 92:33–36.

15 Hyman BT, Landas SK, Ashman RF, et al. Warfarin related purple toe syndrome and cholesterol microembolization. Am J Med 1987; 82:1233–1237.

16 Freedberg RS, Tunick PA, Kronzon I. Emboli in transit: the missing link. J Am Soc Echo 1998; 11:826–828.

17 Amarenco P, Cohen A, Tzourio C, et al. Atherosclerotic disease of the aortic arch and the risk of ischemic stroke. N Engl J Med 1994; 331:1474–1479.

18 Jones EF, Kalman JM, Calafiore P, et al. Proximal aortic atheroma: an independent risk factor for cerebral ischemia. Stroke 1995; 26:218–224.

19 Tunick PA, Rosenzweig BP, Katz ES, et al. High risk for vascular events in patients with protruding aortic atheromas: a prospective study. J Am Coll Cardiol 1994; 23:1085–1090.

20 Amarenco P, Cohen A for the French Study of Aortic Plaques in Stroke Group. Atheroscle-

rotic disease of the aortic arch as a risk factor for recurrent ischemic stroke. N Engl J Med 1996; 334:1216–1221.

21 Stern A, Tunick PA, Culliford AT, *et al*. Protruding aortic arch atheromas: risk of stroke during heart surgery with and without aortic arch endarterectomy. Am Heart J 1999; 138:746–752.

22 Tunick PA, Lackner H, Katz ES, *et al*. Multiple emboli from a large aortic arch thrombus in a patient with thrombotic diathesis. Am Heart J 1992; 124:239–241.

23 Tunick PA, Culliford A, Lamparello P, Kronzon I. Atheromatosis of the aortic arch as an occult source of multiple systemic emboli. Ann Intern Med 1991; 114:391–392.

24 Khatibzadeh M, Mitusch R, Stierle U, *et al*. Aortic atherosclerotic plaque as a source of systemic embolism. J Am Coll Cardiol 1996; 27:664–669.

25 Khandheria BK, Seward JB, Tajik AJ. Transesophageal echocardiography. Mayo Clin Proc 1994; 69:856–863.

26 Erbel R, Engberding R, Daniel W, Roelandt J, Visser C, Rennollet H. Echocardiography in the diagnosis of aortic dissection. Lancet 1989; 1(8636):457–461.

27 Kronzon I, Tunick PA, Riles T, Rosen R. Transesophageal echocardiography in intimal flap fenestration. J Am Soc Echo 2001; 14:934–936.

28 Rosenzweig BP, Goldstein S, Sherrid M, Kronzon I. Aortic dissection with flap prolapse into the left ventricle. Am J Cardiol 1996; 77:214–216.

29 Keren A, Kim CB, Hu BS, *et al*. Accuracy of biplane and multiplane transesophageal echocardiography in diagnosis of typical acute aortic dissection and intramural hematoma. J Am Coll Cardiol 1996; 28:627–636.

30 Nienaber CA, Sievers H-H. Intramural hematoma in acute aortic syndrome: more then one variant of dissection? Circulation 2002; 106:284–285.

6 # Abdominal Aorta Imaging

Emile R. Mohler III

The abdominal aorta is easily visualized with ultrasound via a transcutaneous approach, as opposed to imaging of the thoracic aorta in which air in the intervening lung makes imaging difficult. Diseases of the abdominal aorta that may be identified with ultrasound include atherosclerotic and aneurysmal disease, dissection, and congenital anomalies.

Abdominal aortic aneurysm

Characteristics

An abdominal aortic aneurysm (AAA) is defined as an aortic diameter of at least 1.5 times the diameter measured at the level of the renal arteries. A normal diameter of the abdominal aorta is approximately 2.0 cm (range, 1.4–3.0 cm) in most individuals; a diameter of > 3.0 cm is considered to be aneurysmal[1]. A family history of AAA results in a four-fold increase in the risk of developing this condition[2]. In addition, if an aneurysm is found in one vascular territory, such as the popliteal artery, there is an increased risk of an aneurysm in the aorta.

AAAs are described as saccular, fusiform, or cylindrical (Figure 6.1). The majority of AAAs are fusiform in shape, located below the renal arteries, and may involve one or both of the iliac arteries. Atherosclerotic changes and/or mural thrombus commonly line the aneurysmal sac and may be a source of emboli[3]. Dissection has been reported with AAA; however, this is less common.

Risk factors for the development of an AAA include an older age, smoking, male sex, hypertension, atherosclerosis, family history, and aneurysms in popliteal or femoral arteries[4]. The typical growth rate reported in the literature of AAAs measuring 3–5.9 cm is approximately 0.3–0.4 cm per year[5,6]. However, larger aneurysms may progress more rapidly than others, while some aneurysms may remain dormant and then expand rapidly.

Aortic dissection

Pathophysiology

The pathologic event resulting in aortic dissection is a tear in the aortic intima. The intimal tear may occur as a result of trauma (usually thoracic aorta) or secondary to degeneration of the aortic media (cystic medial necrosis). Blood

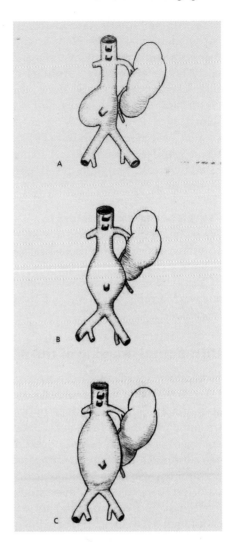

Figure 6.1 Schematic diagram showing the various shapes that an abdominal aortic aneurysm (AAA) may elicit. (A) Saccular, (B) fusiform, (C) cylindrical. Zaccardi MJ, Chapter 22, page 336. In: Strandness DE, Jr. (ed.) *Duplex Scanning in Vascular Disorders*, 3rd edn. Philadelphia: Lippincott, Williams and Wilkins, 2002.

passes through the tear, creating a channel (false lumen) which separates the intimal layer from the surrounding media and/or adventitia.

Classification

Aortic dissections are classified according to one of two anatomic systems: the DeBakey system or the Daily (Stanford) system. The DeBakey system classifies aortic dissection into three types: Type I involves both the ascending and descending thoracic aorta, Type II is confined to the ascending aorta, and Type III is confined to the descending aorta[7]. The Daily system describes aortic dissection involving the ascending aorta as Type A and all other dissections as Type B[8]. One variant of aortic dissection is an intramural hematoma, in which hemorrhage in the aortic wall occurs, presumably from degeneration of the vasovasorum or ruptured atherosclerotic plaque, without an intimal tear[9]. The intima can also tear without resulting hematoma and may only be evidenced by an eccentric aortic bulge on imaging[10]. Another related entity is penetrating aortic ulceration, whereby an ulcerated aortic atherosclerotic lesion penetrates the internal elastic lamina into the media, and is seen as an outpouching of the aortic wall with jagged edges, usually in an area of extensive atheroma, with transesophageal echocardiography (TEE), computed tomography (CT), or magnetic resonance (MR) imaging (see Chapter 5). These aortic ulcers may be complicated by breakthrough to the adventitia, causing a pseudoaneurysm or complete rupture[11].

Prevalence and risk factors

Ascending aortic dissections are estimated to be almost twice as common as descending aortic dissections. Risk factors for the development of aortic dissection include an older age, male gender, and hypertension[12]. Other causes of aortic dissection that may occur in younger individuals are congenital abnormalities, such as Marfan's syndrome and Turner's syndrome, as well as illicit drug use (cocaine)[13].

Ultrasound imaging of the abdominal aorta

Indications for abdominal aortic imaging

Ultrasound imaging is highly sensitive for assessing and following the size of abdominal aneurysms[14]. Major indications for the assessment of AAA with ultrasound imaging include, but are not limited to: abdominal pain; pulsatile and enlarged aorta on physical examination; hemodynamic compromise suggestive of a ruptured aneurysm; an immediate family member with a history of AAA; and an aneurysm found in another vascular territory[15]. Patients with abdominal pain and suspected aortic dissection are also candidates for ultrasound imaging. If a diagnosis of ruptured aorta is entertained, ultrasound or CT imaging should not delay surgical repair, but only be obtained if readily available in the emergency setting. The differential diagnosis of a ruptured or leaking aneurysm may include other acute conditions, such as renal colic, diverticulitis, pancreatitis, inferior wall coronary ischemia, mesenteric ischemia, or biliary tract disease. In addition, elderly patients who present with hypotension from a leaking AAA may have electrocardiographic changes consistent with coronary ischemia.

Abdominal aortic ultrasound imaging technique

The patient is required to fast prior to the study. In order to evaluate an aortoiliac segment, an ultrasound machine with a low-frequency transducer (2.4 MHz) is needed. A mid-range transducer (4–8 MHz) is typically used for femoral or popliteal aneurysms. The examination of an aneurysm should be focused on determining the aneurysm size, shape, location (infra-renal or supra-renal), and distance from other arterial segments.

Ultrasound scanning begins in the supine position. In order to facilitate an accurate measurement of its size, three sonographic views are usually obtained of the abdominal aorta: the sagittal plane (A–P diameter), transverse plane (A–P diameter and transverse diameters), and coronal plane (longitudinal and transverse diameters). Of note, the transducer should be oriented so that the maximal length of the segment is visualized. The transducer is then rotated by 90° to achieve a transverse view. If overlying bowel gas obstructs the aorta from view, patients are instructed to lie in the decubitus position and the aorta is visualized via the coronal plane through either flank. The celiac artery may emerge from the aorta. In addition, the right renal artery may be seen emerging from the aorta and traveling under the inferior vena cava.

Interpretation

A mildly dilated abdominal aorta is described as ectatic when it is > 2.0 cm and < 3.0 cm, whereas it is reported as aneurysmal when the diameter is greater than 3 cm. If an AAA is identified, more information than just the largest diameter should be provided to the referring physician (Table 6.1). The location (proximal, mid-, or distal) and description (saccular, fusiform, or cylindrical) of the AAA are essential (Figure 6.2). The dimensions of the AAA should be reported in the sagittal, transverse, and coronal planes. The presence of a laminated thrombus and/or concomitant atherosclerotic disease is important and should be included in the report. Most abdominal aortic ultrasound evaluations include an evaluation of the iliac arteries, as these may also be aneurysmal. If an endovascular repair is being contemplated, the length of the "neck" at the proximal portion is a critical piece of information. In addition, the tortuosity of the iliac arteries, accessory renal arteries, and calcification of the aortic wall are important when endovascular grafting is being considered. If an abdominal aortic dissection is evident, complete evaluation of the entire aorta is indicated, often using another form of imaging, such as TEE (see Chapter 5), CT, or MR.

Table 6.1 Information for the referring physician when an abdominal aortic aneurysm (AAA) is identified.

Information	Comment
Location of AAA	Proximal, mid-, or distal
Description	Saccular, fusiform, or cylindrical
Dimensions (width and length) in proximal, mid-, and distal sections	Anteroposterior and lateral
Laminated thrombus	Present or absent
Atherosclerotic disease	Present or absent
Calcification of aortic wall	If present, describe extent
Iliac artery aneurysm and/or tortuosity	If present, include dimensions
Accessory renal arteries	Present or absent, especially if aortic stent graft is being considered

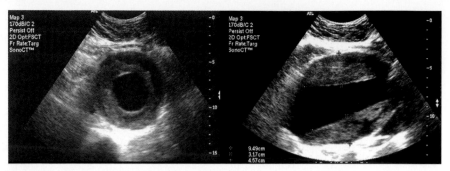

Figure 6.2 Ultrasound image of a fusiform abdominal aortic aneurysm (AAA).

Limitations

The most reliable view for measurement of the abdominal aorta is the anterior posterior view. The lateral view is often the least accurate because of specular reflection artifact (see Chapter 2) from the vessel wall. Hindrances to an adequate examination include overlying bowel gas and obesity, especially in the region of the proximal neck[16]. Thoracic aneurysms are not routinely evaluated with transthoracic ultrasound imaging but are better imaged with TEE (see Chapter 5). Mixed results have been reported for ultrasound follow-up evaluation of aortic endografts. CT angiography is more commonly used for the evaluation of endograft complications, such as endoleak and stent migration[17].

Reference list

1 Ouriel K, Green RM, Donayre C, Shortell CK, Elliott J, DeWeese JA. An evaluation of new methods of expressing aortic aneurysm size: relationship to rupture. J Vasc 1992; 15:12–18.

2 Salo JA, Soisalon-Soininen S, Bondestam S, Mattila PS. Familial occurrence of abdominal aortic aneurysm. Ann Intern Med 1999; 130(8):637–642.

3 Spittell PC, Seward JB, Hallett JW Jr. Mobile thrombi in the abdominal aorta in cases of lower extremity embolic arterial occlusion: value of extended transthoracic echocardiography. Am Heart J 2000; 139(2 Pt 1):241–244.

4 Lederle FA, Johnson GR, Wilson SE, et al. Prevalence and associations of abdominal aortic aneurysm detected through screening. Aneurysm Detection and Management (ADAM) Veterans Affairs Cooperative Study Group. Ann Intern Med 1997; 126(6):441–449.

5 Gadowski GR, Pilcher DB, Ricci MA. Abdominal aortic aneurysm expansion rate: effect of size and beta-adrenergic blockade. J Vasc Surg 1994; 19:727–731.

6 Powell JT, Brady AR. Detection, management, and prospects for the medical treatment of small abdominal aortic aneurysms. Arterioscler Thromb Vasc Biol 2004; 24(2):241–245.

7 DeBakey ME, Henly WS, Cooley DA, Morris GC Jr, Crawford ES, Beall AC Jr. Surgical management of dissecting aneurysms of the aorta. J Thorac Cardiovasc Surg 1965; 49:130–149.

8 Daily PO, Trueblood HW, Stinson EB, Wuerflein RD, Shumway NE. Management of acute aortic dissections. Ann Thorac Surg 1970; 10(3):237–247.

9 Mohr-Kahaly S, Erbel R, Kearney P, Puth M, Meyer J. Aortic intramural hemorrhage visualized by transesophageal echocardiography: findings and prognostic implications. J Am Coll Cardiol 1994; 23(3):658–664.

10 Svensson LG, Labib SB, Eisenhauer AC, Butterly JR. Intimal tear without hematoma: an important variant of aortic dissection that can elude current imaging techniques. Circulation 1999; 99(10):1331–1336.

11 Vilacosta I, Roman JA. Acute aortic syndrome. Heart 2001; 85(4):365–368.

12 Larson EW, Edwards WD. Risk factors for aortic dissection: a necropsy study of 161 cases. Am J Cardiol 1984; 53(6):849–855.

13 Spittell PC, Spittell JA Jr, Joyce JW, *et al*. Clinical features and differential diagnosis of aortic dissection: experience with 236 cases (1980 through 1990). Mayo Clin Proc 1993; 68(7):642–651.

14 LaRoy LL, Cormier PJ, Matalon TA, Patel SK, Turner DA, Silver B. Imaging of abdominal aortic aneurysms. Am J Roentgenol 1989; 152:785–792.

15 Powell JT, Greenhalgh RM. Clinical practice. Small abdominal aortic aneurysms. N Engl J Med 2003; 348(19):1895–1901.

16 Scott RA, Ashton HA, Kay DN. Abdominal aortic aneurysm in 4237 screened patients: prevalence, development and management over 6 years [see comments]. Br J Surg 1991; 78:1122–1125.

17 Wolf YG, Johnson BL, Hill BB, Rubin GD, Fogarty TJ, Zarins CK. Duplex ultrasound scanning versus computed tomographic angiography for postoperative evaluation of endovascular abdominal aortic aneurysm repair. J Vasc Surg 2000; 32(6):1142–1148.

IV Renal and Visceral

7 Renal Artery Duplex Ultrasonography

Michael R. Jaff

Introduction

Although generally believed to be a rare cause of hypertension, atherosclerotic renal artery stenosis (RAS) is a common finding in selected patient populations. In the general population of hypertensive patients, 1–6% have some element of RAS[1]. However, there are several clinical clues which suggest an increased likelihood of RAS in certain patient subsets, including the presence of coronary, carotid, abdominal aortic, and lower extremity peripheral arterial disease. In patients with aorto-iliac or abdominal aortic aneurysmal disease, the prevalence of significant bilateral renal artery disease is in the range 33–45%[2,3].

Coronary artery atherosclerosis is a similar marker for RAS. In 346 patients with aneurysmal or occlusive vascular disease prompting arteriography, 28% had significant RAS. Of the patients with RAS, 58% had clinically overt coronary artery disease. In those patients without RAS, the incidence of coronary artery disease was only 39%[4]. In a prospective study of 1302 patients undergoing coronary arteriography, abdominal aortography demonstrated significant RAS in 15% of patients. The number of coronary arteries involved with atherosclerosis also predicted the likelihood of RAS in this series. For example, if one coronary artery demonstrated atherosclerosis, the prevalence of significant RAS was 10.7%. If three coronary arteries demonstrated atherosclerotic involvement, the prevalence of RAS was 39.0%[5].

The prevalence of unsuspected, significant RAS in patients with renal insufficiency is surprisingly high, up to 24% in one series[6]. The 5 year survival of patients aged 65–74 years with end-stage renal disease (ESRD) due to hypertension was 20%, and was only 9% in patients aged ≥75 years. Of those patients with hypertensive ESRD, 83 of 683 dialysis patients had significant RAS[7]. The 15 year survival of patients with ESRD because of RAS was 0%, compared with 32% for patients on dialysis due to, for example, polycystic kidney disease. In a prospective angiographic trial, RAS was the cause of ESRD in 14% of new patients beginning dialysis[8].

Once RAS is discovered, the clinical course and natural history may help to predict the clinical benefit from revascularization. Although there remains controversy about the true natural history of RAS, in one independent arteriographic series, 39% of patients demonstrated progression of RAS[9]. In a pooled review of five arteriographic trials, 49% of the renal arteries demonstrated progression of stenosis[10]. Fourteen per cent of these vessels progressed to occlusion.

In a retrospective series of 85 patients with RAS followed for a mean of 52 months, 44% demonstrated progression of RAS and 16% demonstrated progression to total occlusion, with progression occurring within the first 2 years in 46% of renal arteries[11]. In the same series, 78 initial renal arteries with <50% stenosis were followed. Of these renal arteries, 69% demonstrated no significant progression of stenosis. However, of 18 renal arteries with baseline stenosis of >75–99%, 39% progressed to occlusion on sequential arteriography. Finally, deterioration in renal function, as measured by an increase in the serum creatinine, occurred in 54% of patients with progressive stenosis of the renal artery, while only 25% demonstrated an increase in serum creatinine when there was no progression of disease ($P < 0.02$). Renal size decreased in 70% of patients with progressive disease, but in only 27% of patients without increasing stenosis ($P < 0.001$).

In one of only two prospective natural history studies of RAS, Dean et al.[12] followed 41 patients with RAS whose treatment was medical, i.e. control of hypertension and correction of any coexisting renal diseases, if possible. Progression of RAS occurred when blood pressure was well controlled; 40% of patients developed an increase in serum creatinine, and 37% of patients demonstrated a decrease in renal mass. The second prospective study involved the use of renal artery duplex ultrasonography (RADUS). In this study, 84 patients with at least one abnormal renal artery, whose therapy did not involve revascularization, were included. Of 139 renal arteries over the course of a mean follow-up of almost 13 months, the progression of RAS, as documented by RADUS, was 42% at 2 years. The occlusion rate at 2 years was 11%. The overall progression rate was 20%[13].

Until recently, the correlation between progressive RAS and deterioration in renal function had not been demonstrated. This is a critical issue, as many patients presently undergo renal artery revascularization in an effort to preserve renal function. Caps et al.[14] have demonstrated that untreated RAS leads to renal atrophy. Of 204 kidneys with varying degrees of RAS in 122 patients, followed for a mean of 33 months, the 2 year incidence of renal atrophy (>1 cm) was 20.8% in patients with severe baseline RAS ($P = 0.009$ compared with normal or mild baseline RAS). A baseline systolic blood pressure of >180 mmHg and duplex ultrasound findings suggestive of significant RAS also predicted a higher likelihood of progressive renal atrophy. Of greatest importance, these data revealed that patients who demonstrated bilateral renal atrophy suffered a greater increase in serum creatinine than patients who were found to have no renal atrophy ($P = 0.03$).

Indications for testing

Patients with resistant or refractory hypertension, malignant hypertension, or unexplained azotemia, all in association with atherosclerosis elsewhere, are candidates for further investigation for RAS.

Noninvasive test options

Although a number of noninvasive methods of diagnosis of RAS have been proposed, none has obviated the role of the "gold standard," renal arteriography. Each "screening" test has significant limitations that prevent widespread acceptance. Plasma renin activity has inadequate sensitivity and specificity to be used as the sole diagnostic test for RAS, even with stimulation with an angiotensin-converting enzyme inhibitor. Captopril-stimulated nuclear renal flow scanning is an accurate screening test for the diagnosis of unilateral RAS in a patient with normal renal function. However, in cases of bilateral RAS, and in patients with impaired renal function, the accuracy of this test decreases, and it cannot be used in screening.

Renal vein renin ratios can be helpful; however, this is an invasive diagnostic test requiring that most, if not all, antihypertensive agents be withdrawn prior to sampling. Given that many of these patients have poorly controlled hypertension, hospitalization and the use of parenteral antihypertensive agents would be required for adequate performance of this test.

RADUS offers many appealing advantages over other diagnostic options. RADUS provides direct visualization of the renal arteries and kidneys, and allows for accurate "surveillance" of revascularization to detect early failure (either surgical or endovascular revascularization).

Several investigators have demonstrated the validity of duplex ultrasonography for the diagnosis of RAS. In one prospective series, 29 patients (58 renal arteries) underwent duplex ultrasonography and contrast arteriography. The sensitivity, specificity, and positive predictive value of RADUS were 84%, 97%, and 94%, respectively, for a detection of > 60% stenosis[15]. Utilizing a peak systolic velocity (PSV) criterion of > 180 cm s^{-1} within the renal artery, duplex scanning was able to distinguish between normal and diseased renal arteries with a sensitivity of 95% and a specificity of 90%[16]. A ratio of PSV in the area of RAS to PSV within the aorta (renal to aortic ratio, RAR) of > 3.5 predicts the presence of > 60% RAS. Using this criterion, renal artery duplex demonstrated a sensitivity of 92%.

In a large prospective series of 102 consecutive patients who underwent both duplex ultrasonography and contrast arteriography within 1 month of each other, 62 of 63 arteries with < 60% stenosis, 31 of 32 arteries with 60–79% stenosis, and 67 of 69 arteries with 80–99% stenosis were correctly characterized by duplex ultrasonography. Occluded renal arteries were correctly identified by ultrasonography in 22 of 23 cases. The overall sensitivity, specificity, positive predictive value, and negative predictive value of duplex ultrasonography were 98%, 99%, 99%, and 97%, respectively[17].

Technique of renal artery duplex ultrasonography

All examinations should be performed after an overnight fast, and many choose to use an oral simethicone-containing product prior to the examination in an

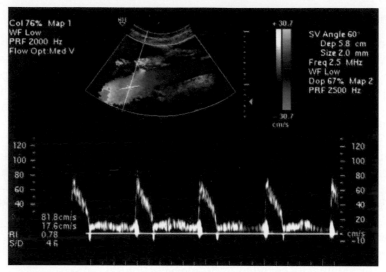

Figure 7.1 Color duplex ultrasound of the abdominal aorta at the level of the renal arteries. The Doppler peak systolic velocity is used as the denominator of the renal to aortic ratio.

effort to reduce gas. Patients may take their medication at the normal time with a sip of water. Renal artery ultrasound should be performed from both an anterior and oblique [or posterior (flank)] approach using a curved array 2.5–3.0 MHz transducer. With a longitudinal (long-axis) view, the flow velocity in the aorta is recorded at the level of the renal arteries (Figure 7.1). This velocity and the highest renal artery PSV are used to calculate RAR. From the anterior approach, key landmarks for orientation include the celiac axis, superior mesenteric artery, and the left renal vein as it crosses anterior to the aorta (Figure 7.2).

The renal arteries are best visualized in a transverse (short-axis) view. Using the B mode image and a Doppler angle of insonation of $\leq 60°$, the arteries are interrogated. The Doppler should be "walked" throughout the entire artery from the origin to the renal hilum. The PSV and end-diastolic velocity are recorded from the renal artery origin, and proximal, mid-, and distal segments. The normal Doppler spectrum in a renal artery is "low resistant," generating persistent diastolic flow (Figure 7.3). From the flank approach, the renal artery can be visualized at the renal hilum and followed to the aorta (Figure 7.4). It is critical that two views are obtained to assure the examiner that the correct Doppler angle of insonation has been used and that a focal increase in systolic velocities has not been missed from one view.

RAR, the ratio of the PSV in the renal arteries to the PSV in the aorta, is used to classify the degree of stenosis. A three-category classification scheme is commonly used: 0–59% stenosis, 60–99% stenosis, and total occlusion. When the aortic velocity is $< 40\,\mathrm{cm\,s^{-1}}$ or $> 100\,\mathrm{cm\,s^{-1}}$, RAR is not an accurate representation of the degree of stenosis. In these instances, if the PSV is $> 200\,\mathrm{cm\,s^{-1}}$ and post-stenotic turbulence is present on color flow, the stenosis is classified as 60–99%

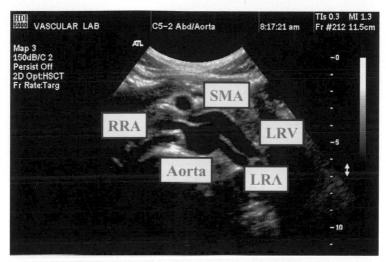

Figure 7.2 A gray scale image identifying the important landmarks for successful renal artery imaging. LRA = left renal artery; LRV = left renal vein; RRA = right renal artery; SMA = superior mesenteric artery. Note the orientation of the SMA to the aorta, as well as the LRV, which crosses anterior to the aorta in 80% of patients. Retroaortic LRVs must be recognized.

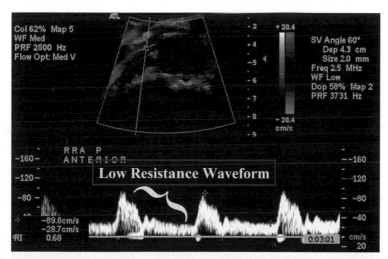

Figure 7.3 Normal Doppler spectral waveform of a renal artery. As the kidney is a "low-resistant" vascular bed, the waveform demonstrates continuous diastolic flow.

(Figure 7.5). When there is a discrepancy in kidney size of 2.0 cm or greater, the ultrasonographer should search very carefully for the presence of RAS or an occluded renal artery.

The acceleration time (AT), acceleration index (AI), and resistive index (RI) have been used by some laboratories to diagnose RAS. These measurements are

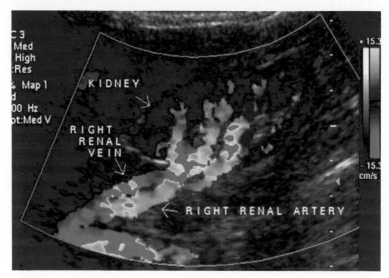

Figure 7.4 Color duplex image obtained from the lateral decubitus position, demonstrating the entire right renal artery from the origin at the aorta into the cortical branches within the kidney.

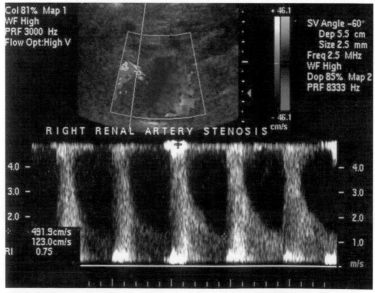

Figure 7.5 Color duplex image of a 60–99% right renal artery stenosis. Note that the Doppler angle is 60° and parallel to the direction of arterial flow. There is a dramatic increase in the peak systolic and end-diastolic velocities, correlating with 60–99% renal artery stenosis.

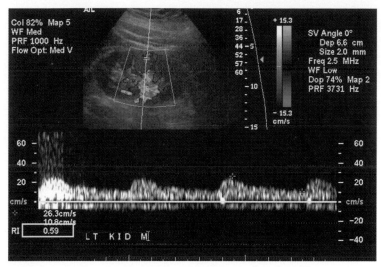

Figure 7.6 Doppler waveform of a cortical branch within the kidney. Note that the waveform was obtained using a 0° Doppler angle. The yellow box identifies the renal resistive index which, in this example, is normal. This demonstrates low resistance within the end organ.

obtained by Doppler examination in the renal parenchyma using an oblique approach. The Doppler measurements are made with a 0° angle in order to obtain the best Doppler waveform possible. AT, measured in milliseconds, is the time from the onset of the upstroke of the arterial wave to the systolic peak. AI is the slope of the acceleration curve. AI < 291 cm s^{-2} suggests a hemodynamically significant stenosis[18].

RI is a measure of the resistance within the renal circulation[19] (Figure 7.6). An elevated RI may be present in renal parenchymal disease as a result of some antihypertensive agents, and due to age[20]. It is not useful for predicting the degree of RAS. However, recent data have suggested that a normal renal RI prior to revascularization predicts a beneficial impact of such revascularization on blood pressure and renal function[21]. The use of the renal RI, AT, and AI should be as correlative values rather than as criteria for RAS in and of themselves.

Duplex ultrasonography is the ideal method of determining the adequacy of revascularization[22]. Given the proliferation of endovascular therapy (percutaneous angioplasty with stent deployment)[23], duplex ultrasonography is helpful in detecting important areas of restenosis within renal artery stents (Figure 7.7). Dean et al.[12] compared angiography with duplex ultrasound for the follow-up of RAS after angioplasty, and demonstrated a sensitivity and specificity of 69% and 98%, respectively, for the detection of stenosis of > 60%. Bakker et al.[24] showed similar results in 33 renal arteries treated with angioplasty followed by stent placement. All patients who have undergone percutaneous intervention should be placed in a surveillance program in an attempt to identify restenosis prior to occlusion.

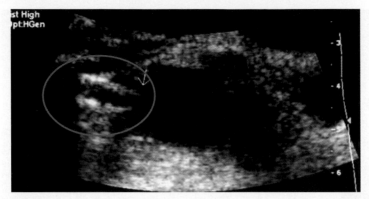

Figure 7.7 Gray scale image of a right renal artery stent. Note that the proximal aspect of the stent is within the aortic lumen, which is ideal positioning. Given that the majority of atherosclerotic plaque in the renal artery is aorto-ostial, covering the aortic plaque is critical to alleviating the hemodynamic impact of the stent.

Limitations

The limitations of RADUS are generally a result of the body habitus and overlying bowel gas seen in patients. If a significant amount of bowel gas is present and obscures views on the initial cursory images, the patient should be invited back on another day for another attempt. Patients must be able to halt respiration on command in order to obtain a representative Doppler spectral waveform at a correct Doppler angle.

The greatest limitation of RADUS is the identification of accessory or "polar" renal arteries. This requires tremendous patience and persistence. If there is a strong clinical suspicion for RAS, and the main renal arteries are patent, further imaging should be considered.

The learning curve for mastering RADUS is steep. The technologist and physician must have hands-on training and proctoring. In addition, when starting the performance of RADUS, adequate time should be allocated, as examinations may take 60–90 min to complete. As experience grows, the examination time shortens, and a skilled technologist often completes an examination in 45 min.

Reference list

1 Simon N, Franklin SS, Bleifer KH, Maxwell MH. Clinical characteristics of renovascular hypertension. J Am Med Assoc 1972; 220:1209–1218.
2 Olin JW, Melia M, Young JR, *et al.* Prevalence of atherosclerotic renal artery stenosis in patients with atherosclerosis elsewhere. Am J Med 1990; 88:46N–51N.
3 Missouris CG, Buckenham T, Cappucio FP, MacGregor GA. Renal artery stenosis: a common and important problem in patients with peripheral vascular disease. Am J Med 1994; 96:10–14.

4 Valentine RJ, Clagett GP, Miller GL, *et al.* The coronary risk of unsuspected renal artery stenosis. J Vasc Surg 1993; 18:433–440.

5 Harding MB, Smith LR, Himmelstein SI, *et al.* Renal artery stenosis: prevalence and associated risk factors in patients undergoing routine cardiac catheterization. J Am Soc Nephrol 1992; 2:1608–1616.

6 O'Neil EA, Hansen KJ, Canzanello VJ, *et al.* Prevalence of ischemic nephropathy in patients with renal insufficiency. Am Surg 1992; 58:485–490.

7 Mailloux LU, Napolitano B, Bellucci AG, *et al.* Renal vascular disease causing end-stage renal disease, incidence, clinical correlates, and outcomes: a 20-year clinical experience. Am J Kidney Dis 1994; 24:622–629.

8 Scoble JE, Maher ER, Hamilton G, *et al.* Atherosclerotic renovascular disease causing renal impairment—a case for treatment. Clin Nephrol 1989; 31.119–122.

9 Meaney TF, Dustan IIP, McCormack LJ. Natural history of renal arterial disease. Radiology 1968; 9:877–887.

10 Greco BA, Breyer JA. The natural history of renal artery stenosis: who should be evaluated for suspected ischemic nephropathy? Semin Nephrol 1996; 16:2–11.

11 Schreiber MJ, Pohl MA, Novick AC. The natural history of atherosclerotic and fibrous renal artery disease. Urol Clin N Am 1984; 11:383–392.

12 Dean RH, Kieffer RW, Smith BM, *et al.* Renovascular hypertension: anatomic and renal function changes during therapy. Arch Surg 1981; 116:1408–1415.

13 Zierler RE, Bergelin RO, Isaacson JA, *et al.* Natural history of atherosclerotic renal artery stenosis: a prospective study with duplex ultrasonography. J Vasc Surg 1994; 19:250–258.

14 Caps MT, Zierler RE, Polissar NL, *et al.* Risk of atrophy in kidneys with atherosclerotic renal artery stenosis. Kidney Int 1998; 53:735–742.

15 Taylor DC, Kettler MD, Moneta GL, *et al.* Duplex ultrasound scanning in the diagnosis of renal artery stenosis: a prospective evaluation. J Vasc Surg 1988; 7:363–369.

16 Strandness DE. Duplex imaging for the detection of renal artery stenosis. Am J Kidney Dis 1994; 24:674–678.

17 Olin JW, Piedmonte MR, Young JR, *et al.* The utility of duplex ultrasound scanning of the renal arteries for diagnosing significant renal artery stenosis. Ann Intern Med 1995; 122:833–838.

18 Isaacson J, Neumyer MM. Direct and indirect renal arterial duplex and Doppler color flow evaluations. J Vasc Technol 1995; 19(5–6):309–316.

19 Kim SH, Kim WH, Choi BI, *et al.* Duplex Doppler US in patients with medical renal disease: resistive index vs. serum creatinine level. Clin Radiol 1992; 45:85–87.

20 Malatino LS, Polizzi G, Garozzo M, *et al.* Diagnosis of renovascular disease by extra- and intrarenal Doppler parameters. Angiology 1998; 49:707–721.

21 Rademacher J, Chavan A, Bleck J, *et al.* Use of Doppler ultrasonography to predict the outcome of therapy for renal-artery stenosis. N Engl J Med 2001; 344:410–417.

22 Eidt JF, Fry RE, Clagett GP, *et al.* Postoperative follow-up of renal artery reconstruction with duplex ultrasound. J Vasc Surg 1988; 8:667–673.

23 Dorros G, Jaff M, Mathiak L, *et al.* Four-year follow-up of Palmaz–Schatz stent revascularization as treatment for atherosclerotic renal artery stenosis. Circulation 1998; 98:642–647.

24 Bakker J, Beutler JJ, Elgersma OEH, *et al.* Duplex ultrasonography in assessing restenosis of renal artery stents. Cardiovasc Intervent Radiol 1999; 22:475–480.

CHAPTER 8

8 Visceral Duplex Ultrasonography

Thanila A. Macedo

Duplex ultrasound is a widely used imaging tool to evaluate the vascular system. It is an attractive modality as a result of its noninvasive nature, cost, availability, and reliability. Of the many applications of Doppler ultrasound in the abdomen, emphasis is placed on the more challenging and controversial uses, including investigation for mesenteric ischemia and Doppler ultrasound of the liver, incorporating the assessment of transjugular intrahepatic portosystemic shunts (TIPSs). For each of these, normal and abnormal findings are reviewed and the diagnostic criteria proposed in the literature are discussed. The reader should expect to learn the most appropriate sonographic criteria and the limitations of Doppler sonography for each of these uses in the abdomen.

Mesenteric duplex

Introduction
The first report on the use of duplex ultrasound of the mesenteric vessels dates back to the mid-1980s[1]. The diagnostic criteria for celiac and superior mesenteric artery (SMA) stenosis were described in 1991[2,3] on the basis of a retrospective comparison of duplex ultrasound and arteriography, and later validated prospectively[4]. Duplex ultrasound is used as a noninvasive tool in the screening of patients with clinical suspicion of chronic mesenteric ischemia. Patients typically present with post-prandial abdominal pain, "fear of food," and significant weight loss. There is a female predominance (78%)[5]. Symptoms occur as a result of the narrowing or occlusion of the arteries with diminished blood flow to the intestines. The most common underlying cause is atherosclerosis and, less frequently, fibromuscular dysplasia or vasculitis. In symptomatic patients, the disease most commonly affects two or three vessels. Rarely (4%), single artery disease is the cause of mesenteric ischemia as a result of the rich collateral network of the intestines[6]. In the appropriate clinical setting, mesenteric arteriography is the traditional modality for establishing the definitive diagnosis and planning appropriate therapy. However, recent advances in technology have made computed tomographic angiography (CTA) and magnetic resonance angiography (MRA) attractive alternatives for minimally invasive imaging of the vascular system. Treatment options include surgical revascularization or endovascular intervention with or without stent deployment.

Indications

The most common indication for mesenteric arterial duplex ultrasound is for the screening of patients with symptoms of chronic mesenteric ischemia. In patients with acute mesenteric ischemia, mesenteric arteriography is the initial diagnostic test in order to establish the diagnosis in a prompt fashion. Duplex ultrasound can be used intra-operatively and during post-operative surveillance of mesenteric revascularization over time. Intra-operative ultrasound is used to detect technical defects that require immediate revision, and optimizes immediate and long-term technical success. There have been reports on the use of Doppler examination of SMA for the evaluation of small bowel disease[7]. However, the availability and established role of computed tomography (CT) and small bowel contrast studies prevail, and the role of ultrasound is questionable.

Technique

Mesenteric duplex ultrasound is a technically challenging examination. In experienced hands, the examination time is usually 15–20 min. Examination success can be maximized with the use of modern equipment, an experienced sonographer, and appropriate patient selection. Patients are instructed to fast for at least 6 h prior to the examination. Food intake results in changes in the Doppler arterial waveform (generally from high to low resistance within SMA), and the established criteria used for the diagnosis of mesenteric artery stenosis are based on examination performed in the fasting state. Another reason for patients to fast is to help avoid bowel gas, which can preclude visualization of the mesenteric vessels. Understanding the normal anatomy and most frequent variants plays an important role in vessel recognition and the appreciation of pathology (Figure 8.1). Common anatomic variations of interest include a replaced right hepatic artery (17–18%), an accessory right hepatic artery (7–8%), a common hepatic artery arising from SMA (2.5%), a common hepatic artery arising directly from the aorta (2–3%), and a common celiacomesenteric trunk (<1%)[8].

The most commonly used transducers are 4 or 6 MHz curved array or 4 MHz phased array. Occasionally, a lower frequency transducer is needed for improved depth of penetration of the ultrasound beam. The examination is performed with the patient in the supine position, and occasionally in the left lateral decubitus position. In the routine scanning protocol, longitudinal gray scale images are obtained of the abdominal aorta in the proximal, mid-, and distal segments.

Pulsed Doppler waveforms are obtained with angle correction ($\leq 60°$). Peak systolic velocity (PSV) measurements are obtained in the aorta near the celiac axis and SMA. Next, the celiac axis is identified, usually in the longitudinal plane. For all the mesenteric arteries, color Doppler imaging is often useful to identify the arteries, and can help to guide sample volume placement for the pulsed Doppler examination. PSV and end-diastolic velocity (EDV) measurements are obtained at the origin of, and for several centimeters within, the celiac

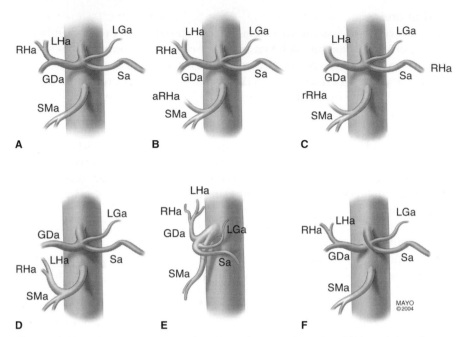

Figure 8.1 Normal and common anatomic variants of mesenteric arteries. (A) Normal: the celiac artery branches are the common hepatic artery, splenic artery, and a small left gastric artery. The superior mesenteric artery arises just inferior to the celiac artery. (B) Accessory right hepatic artery arising from the superior mesenteric artery. (C) Replaced right hepatic artery arising from the superior mesenteric artery. (D) Common hepatic artery arising from the superior mesenteric artery. (E) Common trunk of the celiac and superior mesenteric arteries. (F) Common hepatic artery arising directly from the aorta. aRHa = accessory right hepatic artery; GDa = gastroduodenal artery; LGa = left gastric artery; LHa = left hepatic artery; RHa = right hepatic artery; rRHa = replaced right hepatic artery; Sa = splenic artery; SMa = superior mesenteric artery.

artery. Additional waveforms with PSV and EDV are obtained, first during held deep inspiration and then during held deep exhalation (to exclude the celiac artery compression syndrome). Next, SMA is identified, generally in the longitudinal plane, just inferior to the celiac axis. SMA arises in anterior orientation to the abdominal aorta, and then almost immediately courses in parallel orientation to the aorta for several centimeters. PSV and EDV measurements are obtained at the origin and for several centimeters distally. As SMA courses inferiorly, it can be difficult to obtain a Doppler angle of ≤ 60°, and therefore accurate velocity measurements may only be obtainable from the first few centimeters of SMA. The inferior mesenteric artery (IMA) is a small vessel best identified using the transverse plane a few centimeters above the bifurcation of the aorta. It arises from the left anterolateral aortic wall. PSV and EDV are obtained at the origin and for several centimeters distally, as far as visible. Generally, only a short segment of IMA near the origin can be identified. The course of IMA past the origin can also make it difficult to obtain a Doppler angle of ≤ 60°.

Mesenteric intra-operative duplex ultrasound is a brief examination performed in the surgical suite at the completion of mesenteric revascularization. A variety of transducers (6–8 MHz curved array or 15 MHz linear array) are used, and the probe is placed in a sterile plastic sheath filled with sterile acoustic gel. The abdominal cavity is filled with normal saline. First, using the transverse plane and gray scale, the aorta proximal to the graft, proximal anastomosis, entire length of the graft, distal anastomosis, and native vessel distally are thoroughly evaluated for the presence of technical defects. Next, screening with color Doppler and spectral analysis confirms the absence of hemodynamic disturbance.

When the post-revascularization examination is performed for surveillance, it is helpful to examine the operative report to understand the anatomy of the graft and to review previous examinations, when available. A similar routine is performed with color Doppler images, PSV and EDV obtained in the aorta adjacent to the graft, proximal and distal anastomoses, within the graft (proximal, mid-, and distal), and in the proximal segment of the anastomosed native vessel.

Currently, the use of ultrasound contrast agents is still in development, and does not have an established role. In one study with a small number of patients, there was a tendency towards better visualization and improved diagnosis of significant stenoses in the celiac artery and SMA. It may be helpful in obese patients following mesenteric revascularization or when bowel gas impairs the study[9].

Findings

Normal

In several published series, mesenteric arteries have been successfully identified in 85–100% of patients[4,9,10]. The normal celiac artery and SMA have distinct waveforms reflecting the different end-organ blood supply requirements (Figure 8.2). The major branches of the celiac artery supply the liver and spleen. These organs are low-resistance arterial beds, resulting in a biphasic celiac artery waveform composed of a peak systolic component and higher end-diastolic flow. SMA supplies the small bowel and proximal colon. In the fasting state, when not much blood flow is required by the intestines, the Doppler waveform is triphasic, composed of a systolic peak, an early diastolic reversal of flow, and low end-diastolic flow approaching zero. In the post-prandial state, the end-organ resistance is decreased, and blood flow is increased for adequate food absorption, resulting in changes in the arterial waveform. PSV increases, early diastolic flow reversal disappears, and end-diastolic flow increases. The Doppler arterial waveform is also affected by food composition, with mixed calorie meals resulting in the most pronounced change[11]. A low-resistance waveform can also be a normal finding in SMA in the presence of a replaced (anatomic variant with the right hepatic artery arising from SMA) or accessory (anatomic variant with one right hepatic artery arising from SMA and one from the common hepatic artery/celiac artery) hepatic artery or common hepatic artery arising from SMA (Figure 8.1). Although examination of the IMA is

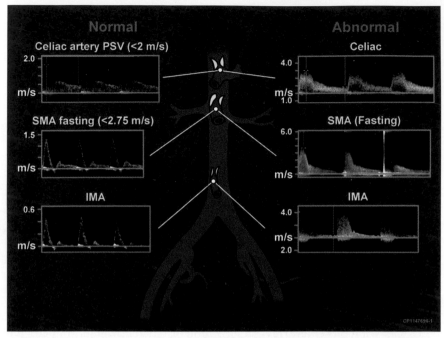

Figure 8.2 Normal and abnormal mesenteric artery Doppler waveforms. The normal celiac artery has a low-resistance waveform. A peak systolic velocity of ≤ 200 cm s^{-1} is indicative of a significant stenosis. The normal superior mesenteric artery has a high-resistance waveform in the post-prandial state and a peak systolic velocity of < 275 cm s^{-1}. The inferior mesenteric artery has a waveform similar to that of the superior mesenteric artery with high resistance.

sometimes considered to be difficult because of its small size and posterior location, it can be identified by skilled sonographers in up to 89% of patients[12]. It supplies the distal colon and upper rectum, and has a high-resistance waveform similar to the triphasic SMA waveform.

A normal intra-operative mesenteric duplex ultrasound is one in which the gray scale images reveal no intraluminal defects and screening color Doppler and spectral waveforms confirm no focally elevated velocities. Nonfocal elevation of velocity can be seen in hyperdynamic states and graft to vessel size mismatch[13]. In this scenario, the absence of post-stenotic turbulence is reassuring.

Post-revascularization duplex ultrasonography can be routinely performed for graft surveillance. It is helpful to have an initial baseline study for future comparison. There are a lack of published data concerning post-revascularization duplex ultrasound. The PSV and waveform are dependent on various factors, such as the size and length of the graft, as well as the type of revascularization: antegrade/retrograde and one- or two-vessel bypass (aorta to celiac and SMA, aorta to SMA, aorta to celiac, or iliac to SMA/celiac). Percutaneous angioplasty and stent placement are relatively recent treatment options for mesenteric ischemia. There is no established protocol or criteria for the surveillance of these patients. In my institution, a baseline study is obtained immediately after the procedure, and thereafter every 6 months, looking for interval increases in velocities indicative of recurrent stenosis.

Abnormal

The diagnostic criteria used to identify mesenteric arterial stenosis at my institution are based on the prospective blind validation study published by Moneta et al.[4]. In this study, a PSV of ≥ 275 cm s^{-1} in SMA and ≥ 200 cm s^{-1} in the celiac artery identified a stenosis of $> 70\%$ with sensitivities of 92% and 87% and specificities of 96% and 80%, respectively (Figure 8.3). The absence of flow is consistent with arterial occlusion unless the examination is technically limited. Other authors have indicated that EDV is more accurate in the detection of SMA stenosis[3,10,14]. An EDV of ≥ 45 cm s^{-1} or no flow signal predicted a SMA stenosis of $\geq 50\%$ or occlusion with an overall accuracy of 91%, sensitivity of 90%, and specificity of 91%; this compared favorably with PSV measurements which, at best, yielded an accuracy of 81%, a sensitivity of 60%, and a specificity of 100%[14]. In the celiac artery, the differences between PSV and EDV did not result in significant changes in accuracy. There are no published validated criteria for IMA stenosis. In our experience (unpublished data), a PSV of ≥ 275 cm s^{-1} (same as the criterion used for SMA) correlates with $\geq 70\%$ stenosis.

Abnormal findings in intra-operative mesenteric duplex are divided into minor and major defects. Minor defects include residual plaque, small intimal

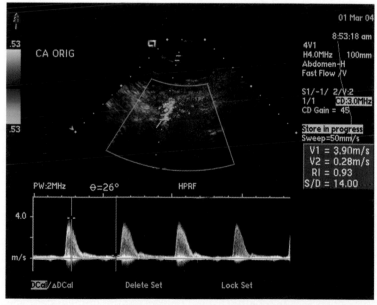

A

Figure 8.3 Doppler ultrasound reveals a peak systolic velocity indicative of a significant stenosis at the origin of the celiac artery (A) and superior mesenteric artery (B). An angiogram (C) confirms the significant stenosis of the celiac (arrow) and superior mesenteric (arrowhead) arteries. *(Continued on p. 90)*

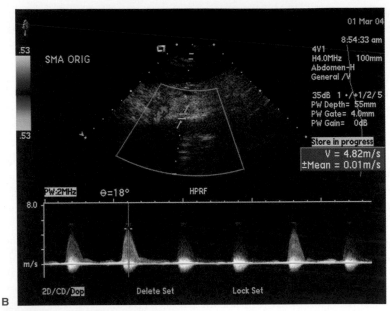

B

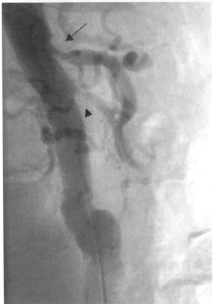

C

Figure 8.3 *Continued*

flap, and graft kinks, which do not result in significant hemodynamic changes and are not necessarily repaired. Major defects require immediate revision and include residual stenosis, thrombus, larger intimal flap, dissection, and bypass graft kinks, which result in significant hemodynamic changes (Figure 8.4)[13]. Post-revascularization duplex ultrasound is used to detect graft patency,

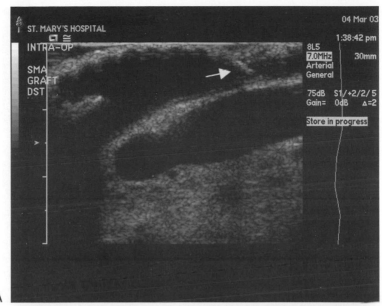

A

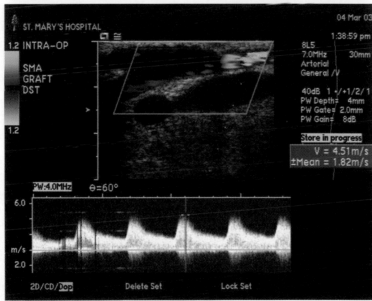

B

Figure 8.4 Intra-operative ultrasound of a supraceliac bifurcated aorta to celiac and superior mesenteric artery bypass graft. (A) Gray scale longitudinal image at the distal anastomosis reveals a linear filling defect (arrow). (B) Spectral Doppler waveform confirms hemodynamic disturbance with an elevated velocity of > 400 cm s^{-1}. A post-surgical revision image reveals the resolution of the intimal flap (C) and the normalization of the velocity (D). *(Continued on p. 92)*

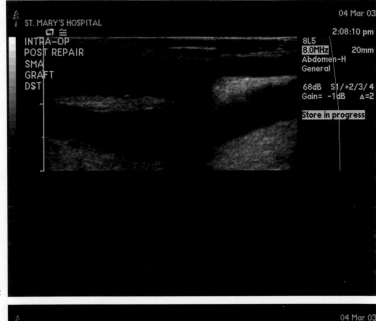

C

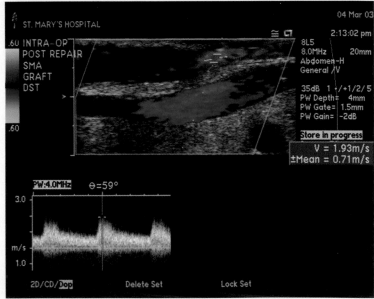

D

Figure 8.4 *Continued*

stenosis, and adjacent fluid collection. Focal elevation of PSV and color mosaic and/or post-stenotic turbulence are suggestive of a significant stenosis (Figure 8.5). Absence of flow is seen in graft occlusion.

The celiac artery compression syndrome is a controversial entity. The celiac

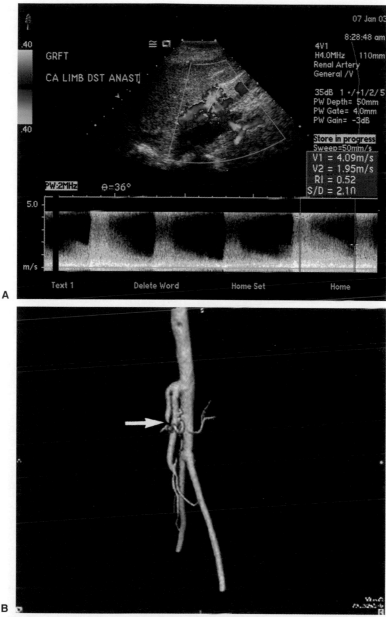

Figure 8.5 Surveillance Doppler ultrasound of a supraceliac bifurcated aorta to celiac and superior mesenteric artery bypass graft. (A) Longitudinal view of the distal celiac limb anastomosis reveals an elevated peak systolic velocity with turbulent flow, indicative of significant stenosis. (B) Computed tomographic angiography with volume-rendered three-dimensional reconstructed image confirms a severe stenosis at the distal anastomosis.

artery is believed to be compressed by the median arcuate ligament of the diaphragm. In inspiration, the celiac artery moves caudally and the arcuate ligament moves ventrally, minimizing compression, while, in expiration, the opposite happens and compression is maximal. The questionable clinical significance of this entity is largely supported by the fact that a significant number of patients have asymptomatic celiac compression[15]. The long-term success of treatment ranges from < 50% to as high as 83%[16,17]. The variations in celiac artery compression related to respiration seen in celiac compression syndrome can be documented with duplex ultrasound. Findings include a significant change in PSV between inspiration and expiration, associated with elevated PSV on expiration (Figure 8.6). There are no established criteria which define significant changes in PSV; however, a doubling of PSV appears to be a reasonable threshold. Ultrasound is used to screen patients prior to confirmatory angiography. Careful interpretation of the ultrasound findings seems prudent; it must be understood that respiratory changes in PSV are seen in patients with celiac compression syndrome, but are not diagnostic.

Limitations

There are many obstacles in mesenteric artery duplex ultrasonography which may account for errors and difficulties in performance and interpretation. These challenges are related to the equipment, operator, patient, or interpretation.

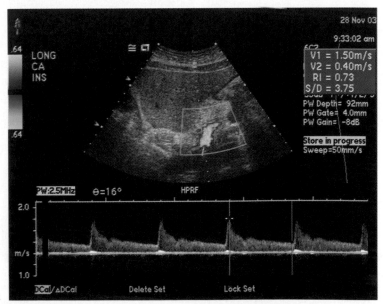

Figure 8.6 Doppler ultrasound of the celiac artery in inspiration (A) reveals a normal peak systolic velocity. In exhalation, the median arcuate ligament of the diaphragm moves superiorly, resulting in compression of the artery and a significant elevation in the peak systolic velocity (B). The lateral aortogram in expiration (C) confirms significant celiac stenosis as a result of compression by the median arcuate ligament.

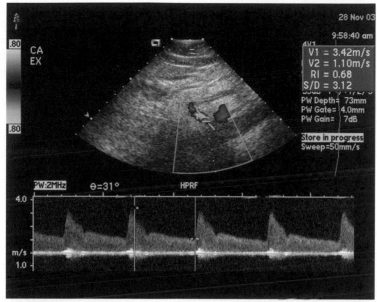

B

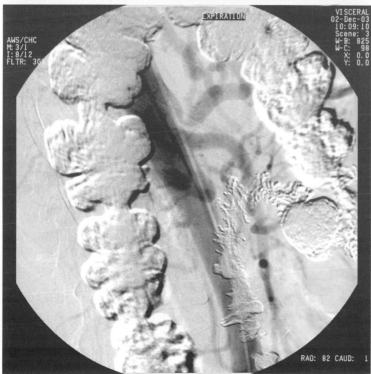

C

Figure 8.6 *Continued*

State-of-the-art equipment and the choice of adequate transducers contribute to a successful examination. The operator's choice of image acquisition parameters, including, but not limited to, the angle of insonation for Doppler sampling, sample volume size, transmit power, filtering, and receiver gain, is important to obtain technically adequate examinations. In experienced hands, these are not limiting factors. Problems may also arise as a result of overlying bowel gas, medications that affect splanchnic vessels (adrenaline, glucagon, vasopressin), changes in central hemodynamics (thyrotoxicosis), or abdominal scars which may limit the acoustic window. Body habitus is also a frequent limiting factor; however, patients with chronic mesenteric ischemia usually present with weight loss. Obesity may raise questions regarding the diagnosis.

Hepatic Doppler

Introduction

Doppler examination is a noninvasive, relatively easy, and inexpensive imaging modality available to evaluate the liver vasculature. It is a routine examination performed in most ultrasound practices. The normal portal and hepatic venous waveform pattern can be affected not only by liver diseases, but also by anomalies in central hemodynamics from other abnormalities (i.e. cardiac). The indications, normal and abnormal findings, and limitations of Doppler sonography of the portal and hepatic veins are reviewed, TIPS is assessed, and liver transplant duplex evaluation is briefly discussed.

Indications

Hepatic Doppler can be used for the evaluation of a wide variety of diseases involving the liver vasculature. The most common indication is for the evaluation of parenchymal liver disease. Patency and the direction of portal venous flow are important pieces of information affecting patients with cirrhosis or chronic hepatitis. In patients with suspected Budd–Chiari syndrome, Doppler ultrasound is useful to confirm impaired hepatic venous outflow. In patients who have undergone bone marrow transplantation, Doppler ultrasound can provide supportive information in the diagnosis of veno-occlusive disease. It is also routinely used to identify vascular complications after hepatic transplantation. Doppler is a useful noninvasive tool to assess the patency and functionality of TIPS. Other uses include the characterization of liver masses and the assessment of portal flow prior to interventions such as hepatic artery embolization. The above indications are not meant to be exhaustive, but exemplify some of the many uses of liver Doppler ultrasound.

Technique

Duplex ultrasound of the liver is usually not a technically challenging examination. The portal and hepatic veins are easily identifiable in most patients, and the examination time is usually no more than 15 min. However, examination of the hepatic artery, especially in immediate post-operative liver transplant patients, can be time consuming and technically challenging. Patients are instructed to fast for at least 6 h prior to the examination, as food intake can affect portal venous flow[18], and bowel gas can obscure extrahepatic vessel analysis. As with any other ultrasound examination, a large body habitus may compromise the study. The most commonly used transducers are 4 or 6 MHz curved array or 4 MHz phased array. Occasionally, a lower frequency transducer is needed for improved depth of penetration of the ultrasound beam. Visualization of the main and right portal veins and right hepatic vein is usually best achieved with the patient in the left posterior oblique or left lateral decubitus position using an intercostal window. The left portal vein and middle and left hepatic veins are best seen with the patient supine through a subcostal approach. When a high left lobe is present, an intercostal window may be better. Pulsed Doppler waveforms are obtained with optimized scanning parameters. In patients in whom Doppler ultrasound is being performed for hepatitis or cirrhosis, velocities and therefore angle correction are not typically needed. When velocities are used to determine the patency of vascular structures (i.e. TIPS), angle correction ($\leq 60°$) is needed. The hepatic veins are sampled near the confluence with the inferior vena cava (IVC), and spectral waveforms are recorded. Waveforms of the main, right, and left portal veins are obtained. Care should be taken to avoid sampling during deep inspiration or expiration because of the effect of these maneuvers on the waveform pattern. In the evaluation of TIPS, color Doppler images of the shunt are obtained. Doppler waveforms are sampled at the portal venous end, mid-shunt, hepatic venous end, main portal vein, and draining hepatic vein. The hepatic artery is routinely evaluated in patients who have undergone hepatic transplantation, or when an abnormality is clinically suspected [aneurysm, arterioportal shunt, or systemic shunt, such as in patients with hereditary hemorrhagic telangiectasia (HHT)]. It can be difficult to identify, and different approaches must be attempted before obtaining an adequate sample. Spectral waveforms of the main, right, and left hepatic arteries are obtained.

Findings

Portal vein

The portal vein is a short vein formed by the splenic and superior mesenteric veins. It bifurcates in right and left branches and follows the hepatic artery and bile duct distribution in the liver parenchyma. It is the major source of blood, accounting for about 75% of the hepatic blood supply. On gray scale images, it can be differentiated from the hepatic veins by the typical echogenic walls. The normal portal vein flow is hepatopetal (i.e. "flow directed towards the liver") with a waveform with minimal phasicity related to respiration and cardiac activity (Figure 8.7A).

Patterns of abnormal portal venous flow are characterized by absent flow, increased waveform phasicity, and/or hepatofugal flow (i.e. "flow away from the liver") (Figure 8.7B–F). Portal vein thrombosis is promptly diagnosed with Doppler sonography (Figure 8.7B). It can be seen as a complication in patients

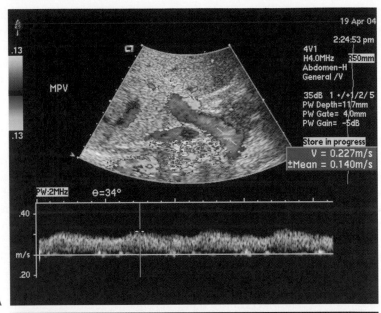

A

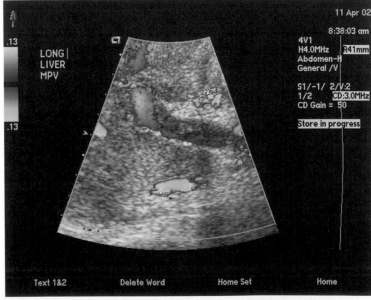

B

Figure 8.7 Patterns of portal vein waveforms on Doppler ultrasound. (A) Normal portal vein waveform with hepatopetal flow and minimal phasicity. (B) Nonocclusive thrombus in the main portal vein in a patient with cirrhosis. (C) Chronic portal vein thrombosis with development of collateral veins in the porta hepatis, also known as "cavernous transformation." (D) Distended main portal vein filled with echogenic thrombus (arrows); spectral Doppler shows arterial flow in the tumor thrombus in a patient with hepatocellular carcinoma. (E) Increased phasicity with a short period of flow reversal in the portal vein as a result of tricuspid regurgitation. (F) Reversal of flow in the main portal vein in a patient with cirrhosis. *(Continued on pp. 99 and 100.)*

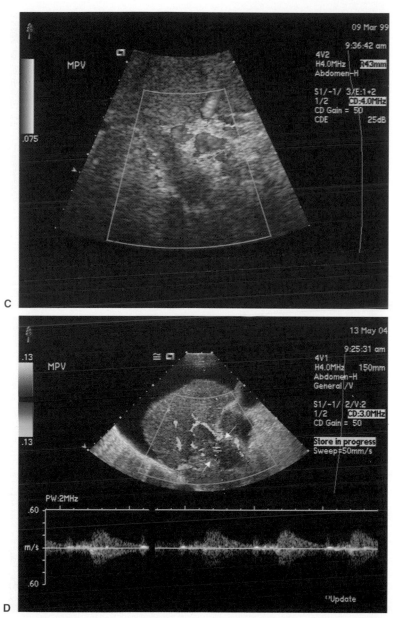

Figure 8.7 *Continued*

with portal hypertension, cirrhosis, hepatitis, pancreatitis, post-splenectomy, liver transplant, trauma, and hypercoagulable states. Long-standing thrombosis leads to the development of multiple collateral veins in the hepatic hilum, with a characteristic appearance known as cavernous transformation of the portal vein (Figure 8.7C). Occasionally, portal venous thrombosis is due to a tumor

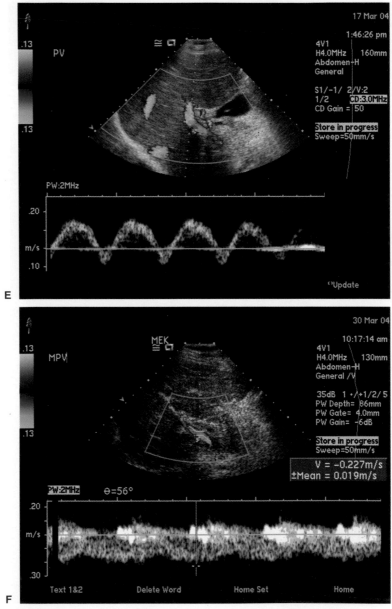

E

F

Figure 8.7 *Continued*

thrombus (Figure 8.7D). The typical finding is of a dilated vein which may have an arterial waveform in the thrombus. Increased phasicity of the portal venous flow (Figure 8.7E) is characterized by exaggeration of the slightly phasic wave-form with wider ranges of PSVs. Although flow is still usually antegrade, occa-sionally there may be a short period of flow reversal. Cardiac and liver diseases are the predominant causes of this abnormality. Increased right atrial pressure results in hepatic venous outflow block with subsequent trans-sinusoidal hepatoportal shunting and transmission of cardiac activity to the portal venous waveform. This phenomenon has been described in patients with tricuspid regurgitation[19], congestive heart failure[20], pulmonary hypertension, constrictive pericarditis[21], mediastinal hematoma, pericardial cyst, right atrial tumor, and pericardial effusion[22]. In patients with liver disease [i.e. cirrhosis, Budd–Chiari syndrome, acute hepatitis, and Caroli's syndrome (combination of congenital hepatic fibrosis and Caroli's disease with cystic and fusiform dilation of the bile ducts)], the development of arterioportal shunts related to sinusoidal outflow obstruction contributes to the increased portal phasicity[23]. Other proposed contributing factors include pulsatile portal venous inflow, transmission of pulsations from the adjacent IVC, and the location of sample volume relative to the IVC[24].

Other uncommon causes of abnormal portal vein pulsatility include arterioportal shunts, seen in HHT or Osler–Weber–Rendu syndrome (a genetic disorder characterized by epistaxis, cutaneous telangiectasia, and visceral arteriovenous malformations), traumatic and iatrogenic causes (prior percutaneous liver biopsy and percutaneous biliary interventions), and portosystemic shunts. It is important to recognize that increased pulsatility of portal venous flow is not always pathologic and can be seen in healthy young adults, especially thin subjects[25].

The other valuable information obtained from portal vein Doppler evaluation is the direction of flow, which has clinical relevance and prognostic implications in patients with liver disease. The reversal of portal venous flow (Figure 8.7F) is indicative of portal hypertension in patients with cirrhosis. It can also occur in patients with Budd–Chiari syndrome or hepatic veno-occlusive disease. Flow reverses when the intrahepatic pressure exceeds that of the portosystemic collateral pathways. Arterioportal communications develop in response to increased resistance to blood inflow. The arterial flow decompresses into the portal vein, resulting in flow reversal to reach the systemic circulation through portosystemic collaterals[26]. Less commonly, the reversal of flow is related to the development of an arterioportal fistula as a result of percutaneous procedures, a focal hepatic lesion, congenital arterial aneurysms, and, rarely, rupture of a hepatic artery aneurysm into the portal vein[27]. Bidirectional flow (to-and-fro) can precede complete flow reversal in cirrhotic patients[28].

Hepatic veins

The hepatic veins drain blood from the liver and join the IVC just before it crosses the diaphragm to enter the right atrium. There are three main hepatic veins: right, middle, and left. Occasionally, accessory veins may be seen, especially those draining the right hepatic lobe. In normal conditions, the small veins draining the caudate lobe directly into the IVC are not seen. The hepatic veins demonstrate a triphasic Doppler waveform reflecting cardiac activity: a biphasic component of forward flow reflecting ventricular systole and diastole, separated by decreased forward flow (or even flow reversal) related to tricuspid closure with atrial overfilling (v wave), followed by a short period of reversed flow reflecting atrial contraction in late diastole (a wave) (Figure 8.8A).

Abnormal hepatic venous waveforms reflect hepatic or cardiac disease, outflow obstruction, and (rarely) anomalous vascular communications. In cirrhosis, decreased phasicity and loss of flow reversal or the finding of a monophasic hepatic venous waveform is observed in 50–75% of patients[29,30]. Hepatic venous outflow obstruction in Budd–Chiari syndrome results in either absent (Figure 8.8B) or monophasic flow in the main hepatic veins. Other findings include narrowing of the hepatic veins, visualization of intrahepatic collateral veins, identification of a caudate vein 3 mm or larger in diameter, and compensatory hypertrophy of the caudate lobe[31,32].

In veno-occlusive disease, a disorder seen in patients on chemotherapy after bone marrow transplantation, loss of the triphasic waveform pattern (similar to Budd–Chiari syndrome) is found, although the obstruction occurs at the sinusoidal level and the main hepatic veins remain patent[33]. The pathophysiologic mechanism of decreased hepatic vein phasicity is related to impaired hepatic venous outflow and altered compliance of the liver parenchyma.

Because of the close proximity of the heart and hepatic veins, cardiac-related hemodynamic changes are promptly reflected in the hepatic venous waveform. Tricuspid regurgitation is responsible for an abnormal hepatic vein waveform, characterized by either decreased or reversed flow during ventricular systole[19]. In constrictive pericarditis, a W-shaped waveform, as a result of reversal of flow in late systole and diastole, has been described[21,34]. Dilation of the hepatic veins and IVC is a sign associated with congestive heart failure. Chronic passive sinusoidal congestion may result in cardiac cirrhosis and a monophasic, low-velocity pattern[35]. Less commonly, abnormalities in the hepatic venous waveform may be related to vascular shunts between either the hepatic artery or portal vein.

Arteriohepatic venous shunts are characterized by an arterialized waveform in the hepatic vein and a low resistive index (RI = PSV – EDV/PSV) in the feeding artery. These can be seen in association with Osler–Weber–Rendu syndrome, cavernous lymphangiomatosis[36], neoplasia, and traumatic or iatrogenic causes[33].

Finally, the interpretation of the abnormal waveform pattern needs to be taken in the context of the clinical presentation as, in certain nonpathologic situations (such as deep inspiration, Valsalva maneuver, and pregnancy), decreased phasicity of the hepatic venous waveform can be found[18,37,38].

Transjugular intrahepatic portosystemic shunt

TIPS is used in the treatment of symptomatic portal hypertension. Most common indications include variceal bleed with failed endoscopic/pharmacologic therapy and recurrent ascites. As described in the name, access to the hepatic vein is gained through a transjugular approach and, with the use of catheters and special devices, a communication is created and a stent is placed between

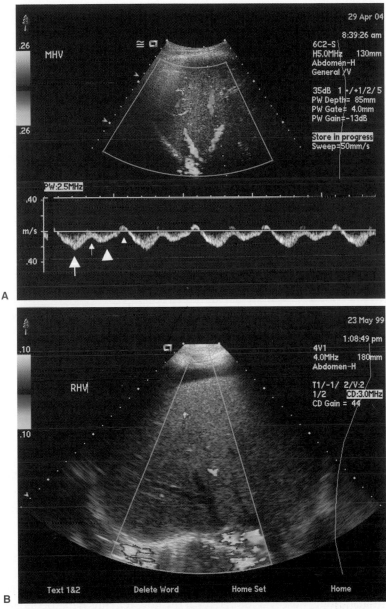

Figure 8.8 (A) Doppler ultrasound of a normal triphasic hepatic vein waveform: biphasic component with forward flow reflecting ventricular systole (large arrow) and diastole (large arrowhead), separated by decreased forward flow (or even flow reversal) related to tricuspid closure and atrial overfilling (v wave, small arrow), followed by a short period of reversed flow (small arrowhead) reflecting atrial contraction. (B) Color Doppler shows the absence of flow in the right hepatic vein in a patient with Budd–Chiari syndrome. (Figure 8.8B provided courtesy of Dr Carl Reading, Mayo Clinic Department of Radiology, Rochester, MN 55905.)

the hepatic vein and portal vein to divert blood from the liver circulation. The primary patency rates range from 25% to 66%[39-41].

The post-procedure evaluation of TIPS includes assessment for patency of the shunt and for evidence of shunt or hepatic vein stenosis. The terms proximal and distal in TIPS have been used variably but, as used here, distal refers to the end of the TIPS that is nearer the hepatic vein. The criteria for the detection of TIPS malfunction are the subject of controversy, and the ideal parameters are yet to be established. The proposed criteria include the maximum and minimum stent PSV, velocity gradient in the stent, main portal vein velocity, temporal change in peak stent velocity and portal vein/hepatic artery velocity, direction of flow in right and left portal vein, and flow direction in the hepatic vein distal to the stent. A wide variability of velocities in normal shunts has been reported. Most of the studies have been performed with the patient in the fasting state. Initial reports evaluated for diminished flow velocities[42-45] described PSV < 50–60 cm s^{-1} as predicting significant stenosis. Other investigators found a poor performance of these low-velocity criteria in the identification of stenosis[42,46,47]. A PSV of 90 cm s^{-1} has been suggested to be a better "lower threshold."[47] A temporal change in the peak stent velocity of > 50 cm s^{-1} between studies was found to be more useful than a single velocity value[48]. Temporal changes in main portal venous velocity of 20–33% have also been described to be indicative of shunt malfunction[47]. The normal mean main portal venous velocity has been reported to be 41–43 cm s^{-1}.[43,44] A main portal venous velocity of < 30 cm s^{-1} has been reported to demonstrate 82% sensitivity and 77% specificity for shunt malfunction[47].

Another proposed strategy is to search for an elevated PSV in the stenotic segment of the stent. PSVs in normal TIPS are variable but can reach 185–220 cm s^{-1}.[45,49,50] A difference between the maximum and minimum stent velocities of > 100 cm s^{-1} was found to have a high positive predictive value but a low sensitivity[47]. The evaluation of multiple parameters predicting TIPS dysfunction found two objective features to be most useful: a main portal vein peak velocity of < 30 cm s^{-1} and an abnormal peak velocity within the distal stent (defined as either < 90 or > 220 cm s^{-1}). When either velocity parameter was abnormal, the sensitivity was 94% and the specificity was 72% and, when both were abnormal, the sensitivity was 55% and the specificity was 100%.

Other potentially useful signs of shunt stenosis include a change from hepatofugal flow (on baseline post-TIPS study) to hepatopetal flow in the right or left portal vein on subsequent scans[45,49,50]. Such a change in flow direction seems to be a late finding, however; moreover, if the flow remains hepatopetal immediately post-TIPS, this sign is not useful.

Reversed flow (away from the IVC) in the draining hepatic vein can be a sign of hepatic vein stenosis[43]. Hepatic artery velocity and RI were not helpful in distinguishing between normal and abnormal shunts[47]. Controversy remains about which Doppler features best predict stenosis. As more data are reported, the ultrasound strategies may change.

Currently, in my institution, we try to obtain a baseline scan within a few days after TIPS placement and then follow the portal vein and shunt velocities (Figure 8.9), also assessing for a temporal change in velocity compared with baseline (> 40 cm s^{-1} decrease or > 60 cm s^{-1} increase). It is important to ensure that the patient has been fasting for at least 6 h, as the velocity in the portal vein and TIPS may increase after eating. If the patient has not been fasting, velocities can spuriously increase and a velocity change could be meaningless.

Liver transplant

Doppler examination of liver transplant patients is a valuable tool to assess for vascular complications. Assessment of hepatic artery patency and anastomotic stenosis is of paramount importance in these patients in whom the hepatic artery represents the sole blood supply to the biliary system. Focally elevated velocity at the anastomosis site of ≥ 200 cm s^{-1}, associated with turbulent flow, is indicative of stenosis (Figure 8.10A). In the early post-operative period, elevated velocity may be related to anastomotic edema and may resolve in subsequent examinations. Unfortunately, visualization of the anastomotic site is frequently difficult, precluding the reliability of this criterion.

Indirect findings, such as the presence of a parvus/tardus waveform distal to the arterial lesion (RI < 0.5 and systolic acceleration time > 0.08 s), have been found to be more accurate for the diagnosis of arterial anastomotic stenosis (Figure 8.10B)[45,48,49]. Elevation of the RI (> 0.75) may be a normal finding soon after hepatic transplantation. However, if the PSV is markedly diminished (< 20 cm s^{-1}), impending thrombosis should be considered. Over time, an elevated RI may be indicative of parenchymal abnormality or transplant rejection. The portal vein is identified to document patency. Focal elevated velocity at the anastomosis with turbulent flow suggests stenosis. Occasionally, echogenic material consistent with thrombus (either occlusive or nonocclusive) is seen in the portal vein. Hepatic vein stenosis is an uncommon vascular complication, found in living donor hepatic transplants. A monophasic hepatic vein waveform is suggestive of the diagnosis, although this finding is not specific[50].

Limitations

Doppler examination of the hepatic and portal vein is not a technically challenging examination in experienced hands. As previously described for mesenteric arterial duplex ultrasonography, the same basic technical principles related to equipment and image acquisition parameters apply. Patient anatomy may occasionally limit the examination, such as when the left lobe of the liver is anatomically cephalad, making visualization challenging. The examination may also be limited in obese patients or when there is a small, cirrhotic liver. In early post-operative patients, an inability to cooperate with breath holding may interfere with waveform sampling, and overlying dressings and subcutaneous scar tissue can limit the acoustic window and the visualization of vessels. In TIPS evaluation, where covered stents with polytetrafluoroethylene (PTFE) fabric

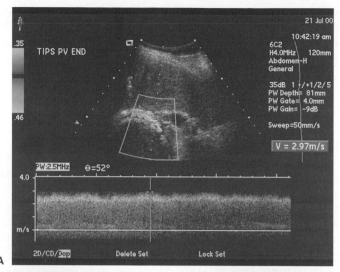

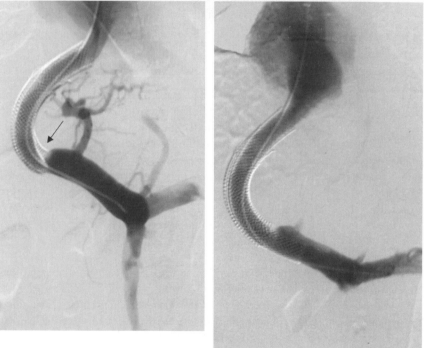

Figure 8.9 (A) Doppler ultrasound reveals elevated velocity (290 cm s^{-1}) at the portal venous end of the transjugular intrahepatic portosystemic shunt (TIPS), consistent with a stenosis. (B) Portal venogram through transjugular access confirms the narrowing at the portal venous end of the TIPS (arrow). (C) Widely patent TIPS after successful balloon dilation of the stenosis.

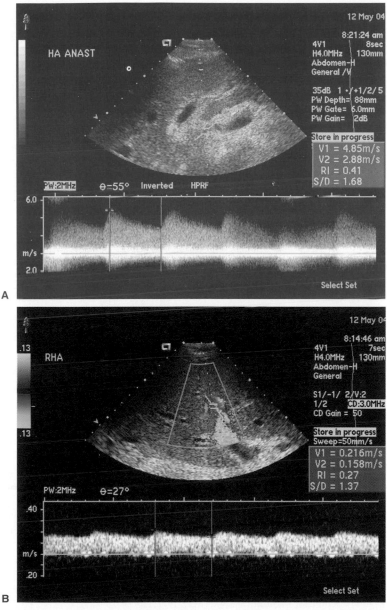

Figure 8.10 (A) Liver transplant Doppler ultrasound of the hepatic artery reveals turbulent flow with elevated peak systolic velocity (480 cm s⁻¹) at the level of the anastomosis, consistent with a stenosis. (B) Tardus/parvus waveform in the right hepatic artery distal to the stenosis.

are used, shadowing within the stent due to embedded gas in the graft fabric may be a problem in the initial post-deployment period.

Reference list

1 Jager KA, Fortner GS, Thiele BL, Strandness DE. Noninvasive diagnosis of intestinal angina. J Clin Ultrasound 1984; 12(9):588–591.

2 Moneta GL, Yeager RA, Dalman R, Antonovic R, Hall LD, Porter JM. Duplex ultrasound criteria for diagnosis of splanchnic artery stenosis or occlusion. J Vasc Surg 1991; 14:511–520.

3 Bowersox JC, Zwolak RM, Walsh DB, *et al.* Duplex ultrasonography in the diagnosis of celiac and mesenteric artery occlusive disease. J Vasc Surg 1991; 14(6):780–786; discussion 786–788.

4 Moneta GL, Lee RW, Yeager RA, Taylor LM Jr, Porter JM. Mesenteric duplex scanning: a blinded prospective study. J Vasc Surg 1993; 17:79–86.

5 Park WM, Cherry KJ, Chua HK, *et al.* Current results of open revascularization for chronic mesenteric ischemia: a standard for comparison. J Vasc Surg 2002; 35(5):853–859.

6 Cho JS, Carr JA, Jacobsen G, Shepard AD, Nypaver TJ, Reddy DJ. Long-term outcome after mesenteric artery reconstruction: a 37-year experience. J Vasc Surg 2002; 35(3):453–460.

7 Britton I, Maguire C, Adams C, Russell RI, Leen E. Assessment of the role and reliability of sonographic post-prandial flow response in grading Crohn's disease activity. Clin Radiol 1998; 53(8):599–603.

8 Kadir SLC, Saeed M. Celiac, superior, and inferior mesenteric arteries. In: Kadir S (ed.), Atlas of Normal and Variant Angiographic Anatomy, p. 299. Philadelphia: W. B. Saunders, 1991.

9 Blebea J, Volteas N, Neumyer M, *et al.* Contrast enhanced duplex ultrasound imaging of the mesenteric arteries. Ann Vasc Surg 2002; 16(1):77–83.

10 Perko MJ, Just S, Schroeder TV. Importance of diastolic velocities in the detection of celiac and mesenteric artery disease by duplex ultrasound. J Vasc Surg 1997; 26(2):288–293.

11 Moneta GL, Taylor DC, Helton WS, Mulholland MW, Strandness DE Jr. Duplex ultrasound measurement of postprandial intestinal blood flow: effect of meal composition. Gastroenterology 1988; 95(5):1294–1301.

12 Mirk P, Palazzoni G, Controneo AR, di Stasi C, Fileni A. Sonographic and Doppler assessment of the inferior mesenteric artery: normal morphologic and hemodynamic features. Abdominal Imaging 1998; 23(4):364–369.

13 Oderich GS, Panneton JM, Macedo TA, *et al.* Intraoperative duplex ultrasound of visceral revascularizations: optimizing technical success and outcome. J Vasc Surg 2003; 38(4): 684–691.

14 Zwolak RM, Fillinger MF, Walsh DB, *et al.* Mesenteric and celiac duplex scanning: a validation study. J Vasc Surg 1998; 27(6):1078–1087; discussion 1088.

15 Levin DC, Baltaxe HA. High incidence of celiac axis narrowing in asymptomatic individuals. Am J Roentgenol, Radium Ther Nucl Med 1972; 116(2):426–429.

16 Evans WE. Long-term evaluation of the celiac band syndrome. Surgery 1974; 76(6):867–871.

17 Lord RS, Tracy GD. Coeliac artery compression. Br J Surg 1980; 67(8):590–593.

18 Teichgraber UKM, Gebel M, Benter T, Manns MP. Effect of respiration, exercise, and food intake on hepatic vein circulation. J Ultrasound Med 1997; 16(8):549–554.

19 Abu-Yousef MM, Milam SG, Farner RM. Pulsatile portal vein flow: a sign of tricuspid regurgitation on duplex Doppler sonography. Am J Roentgenol 1990; 155(4):785–788.

20 Duerinckx AJ, Grant EG, Perrella RR, Szeto A, Tessler FN. The pulsatile portal vein in cases

of congestive heart failure: correlation of duplex Doppler findings with right atrial pressures. Radiology 1990; 176:655–658.

21 Gorka TS, Gorka W. Doppler sonographic diagnosis of severe portal vein pulsatility in constrictive pericarditis: flow normalization after pericardiectomy. J Clin Ultrasound 1999; 27(2):84–88.

22 Gorg C, Riera-Knorrenschild J, Dietrich J. Pictorial review: Colour Doppler ultrasound flow patterns in the portal venous system. Br J Radiol 2002; 75(899):919–929.

23 Gorka W, Gorka TS, Lewall DB. Doppler ultrasound evaluation of advanced portal vein pulsatility in patients with normal echocardiograms. Eur J Ultrasound 1998; 8(2): 119–123.

24 Wachsberg RH, Needleman L, Wilson DJ. Portal vein pulsatility in normal and cirrhotic adults without cardiac disease. J Clin Ultrasound 1995; 23(1):3–15.

25 Gallix BP, Taourel P, Dauzat M, Bruel JM, Lafortune M. Flow pulsatility in the portal venous system: a study of Doppler sonography in healthy adults. Am J Roentgenol 1997; 169(1):141–144.

26 Wachsberg RH, Bahramipou P, Sofocleous CT, Barone A. Hepatofugal flow in the portal venous system: pathophysiology, imaging findings, and diagnostic pitfalls. Radiographics 2002; 22(1):123–140.

27 Vauthey JN, Tomczak RJ, Helmberger T, et al. The arterioportal fistula syndrome: clinicopathologic features, diagnosis, and therapy. Gastroenterology 1997; 113(4):1390–1401.

28 Ralls PW. Color Doppler sonography of the hepatic artery and portal venous system.[see comment]. Am J Roentgenol 1990; 155(3):517–525.

29 Bolondi L, Li Bassi S, Gaiani S, et al. Liver cirrhosis: changes of Doppler waveform of hepatic veins [erratum appears in Radiology 1991; 100(2):586]. Radiology 1991; 178(2):513–516.

30 Colli A, Cocciolo M, Riva C, et al. Abnormalities of Doppler waveform of the hepatic veins in patients with chronic liver disease: correlation with histologic findings. Am J Roentgenol 1994; 162(4):833–837.

31 Chawla Y, Kumar S, Dhiman RK, Suri S, Dilawari JB. Duplex Doppler sonography in patients with Budd–Chiari syndrome. J Gastroenterol Hepatol 1999; 14(9):904–907.

32 Bargallo X, Gilabert R, Nicolau C, Garcia-Pagan JC, Bosch J, Bru C. Sonography of the caudate vein: value in diagnosing Budd–Chiari syndrome. Am J Roentgenol 2003; 181(6):1641–1645.

33 Desser TS, Sze DY, Jeffrey RB. Imaging and intervention in the hepatic veins. Am J Roentgenol 2003; 180(6):1583–1591.

34 von Bibra H, Schober K, Jenni R, Busch R, Sebening H, Blomer H. Diagnosis of constrictive pericarditis by pulsed Doppler echocardiography of the hepatic vein. Am J Cardiol 1989; 63(7):483–488.

35 Gore RM, Mathieu DG, White EM, Ghahremani GG, Panella JS, Rochester D. Passive hepatic congestion: cross-sectional imaging features. Am J Roentgenol 1994; 162(1):71–75.

36 Bodner G, Peer S, Karner M, et al. Nontumorous vascular malformations in the liver: color Doppler ultrasonographic findings. J Ultrasound Med 2002; 21(2):187–197.

37 Roobottom CA, Hunter JD, Weston MJ, Dubbins PA. Hepatic venous Doppler waveforms: changes in pregnancy. J Clin Ultrasound 1995; 23(8):477–482.

38 Abu-Yousef MM. Normal and respiratory variations of the hepatic and portal venous duplex Doppler waveforms with simultaneous electrocardiographic correlation. J Ultrasound Med 1992; 11(6):263–268.

39 LaBerge JM, Ring EJ, Gordon RL, et al. Creation of transjugular intrahepatic portosystemic shunts with the wallstent endoprosthesis: results in 100 patients. Radiology 1993; 187(2):413–420.

40 Lind CD, Malisch TW, Chong WK, *et al.* Incidence of shunt occlusion or stenosis following transjugular intrahepatic portosystemic shunt placement [see comment]. Gastroenterology 1994; 106(5):1277–1283.

41 Haskal ZJ, Pentecost MJ, Soulen MC, Shlansky-Goldberg RD, Baum RA, Cope C. Transjugular intrahepatic portosystemic shunt stenosis and revision: early and midterm results. Am J Roentgenol 1994; 163(2):439–444.

42 Murphy TP, Beecham RP, Kim HM, Webb MS, Scola F. Long-term follow-up after TIPS: use of Doppler velocity criteria for detecting elevation of the portosystemic gradient. J Vasc Intervent Radiol 1998; 9(2):275–281.

43 Surratt RS, Middleton WD, Darcy MD, Melson GL, Brink JA. Morphologic and hemodynamic findings at sonography before and after creation of a transjugular intrahepatic portosystemic shunt. Am J Roentgenol 1993; 160:627–630.

44 Foshager MC, Ferrall H, Nazarian GK, Castañeda-Zuñiga WR, Letourneau JG. Duplex sonography after transjugular intrahepatic portosystemic shunts (TIPS): normal hemodynamic findings and efficacy in predicting shunt patency and stenosis. Am J Roentgenol 1995; 165:1–7.

45 Dodd GD 3rd, Memel DS, Zajko AB, Baron RL, Santaguida LA. Hepatic artery stenosis and thrombosis in transplant recipients: Doppler diagnosis with resistive index and systolic acceleration time. Radiology 1994; 192(3):657–661.

46 Dodd GD, Zajko AB, Orons PD, Martin MS, Eichner LS, Santaguida LA. Detection of transjugular intrahepatic portosystemic shunt dysfunction: value of duplex Doppler sonography. Am J Roentgenol 1995; 164:1119–1124.

47 Kanterman RY, Darcy MD, Middleton WD, Sterling KM, Teefey SA, Pilgram TK. Doppler sonography findings associated with transjugular intrahepatic portosystemic shunt malfunction. Am J Roentgenol 1997; 168:467–472.

48 Platt JF, Yutzy GG, Bude RO, Ellis JH, Rubin JM. Use of Doppler sonography for revealing hepatic artery stenosis in liver transplant recipients. Am J Roentgenol 1997; 168(2):473–476.

49 Vit A, De Candia A, Como G, Del Frate C, Marzio A, Bazzocchi M. Doppler evaluation of arterial complications of adult orthotopic liver transplantation. J Clin Ultrasound 2003; 31(7):339–345.

50 Ko EY, Kim TK, Kim PN, Kim AY, Ha HK, Lee MG. Hepatic vein stenosis after living donor liver transplantation: evaluation with Doppler US. Radiology 2003; 229(3):806–810.

V Extremity Arterial

PART 4
Extremity Animal

9 Segmental Pressures and Pulse Volume Recordings

Emile R. Mohler III

The goals of noninvasive testing for peripheral arterial disease (PAD) are to confirm a suspected diagnosis and to evaluate the level and extent of the arterial obstruction. A variety of arterial studies are used to noninvasively diagnose PAD in the vascular laboratory. Some of these include the combination of segmental limb pressures and pulse volume recordings (plethysmography), exercise treadmill testing, and arterial ultrasonography. Arterial ultrasonography is reviewed in Chapter 10.

Indications for lower extremity noninvasive testing

The major indications for noninvasive assessment of PAD include, but are not limited to, exercise-related limb pain (claudication symptoms), limb pain at rest, extremity ulcer/gangrene, assessment of ischemic wound healing potential, absent peripheral pulses, digital cyanosis, cold sensitivity, arterial trauma and aneurysms, and an abnormal ankle brachial index (see Appendix 1 for ICD-9 and CPT codes). Follow-up evaluation is warranted for surgical bypass graft surveillance, a change in claudication symptoms, and assessment of endovascular revascularization therapy. The contraindications to the performance of segmental pressures and pulse volume recordings include suspected or known deep venous thrombosis, a recent surgical procedure, ulcer, and a cast or bandage that does not allow for compression or should not be compressed with a pneumatic cuff.

The Intersocietal Accreditation of Vascular Laboratories (ICAVL) guidelines indicate that the reporting of PAD must be standardized in the vascular laboratory. Physicians interpreting the noninvasive peripheral vascular examinations must agree on and utilize uniform diagnostic criteria and a standardized report format. Furthermore, details such as the identity of the technician performing the examination must appear as part of the permanent record, and a permanent record of the interpretation must be made available and retained in accordance with applicable standards for medical records.

Segmental limb pressure and pulse volume recording technique

Segmental limb pressure technique

The simplest method for the assessment of PAD in the legs is to measure the ankle/brachial index (ABI), which can be performed in the office setting[1]. The systolic pressures in the brachial arteries of both arms, as well as in the dorsalis pedis and posterior tibial arteries at the ankle level bilaterally, are measured using a hand-held Doppler probe. The ABI for each leg is calculated using the higher of the two arm pressures as the denominator for both the right and left ABI. The higher of the dorsalis pedis and posterior tibial pressures is used as the numerator for the right and left ABI, respectively (Figure 9.1). An abnormal ABI indicates that occlusive arterial disease is present. An abnormal ABI is also a powerful predictor of cardiovascular events[2]. ABI ≤ 0.90 indicates that arterial obstruction is present, and ABI < 0.40 indicates advanced ischemia. An ABI > 1.3 is "supranormal" and indicative of possible medial artery calcification. Patients with supranormal lower extremity pressures are also thought to be at high risk for cardiovascular events[3], and should not be mistaken for having normal peripheral arterial circulation.

The measurement of the ABI does not allow for the assessment of the level of PAD. Obtaining pressures at multiple levels (segmental) in both legs in the vascular laboratory will allow for the further determination of the segment of the artery involved. The evaluation of a segmental pressure gradient between the

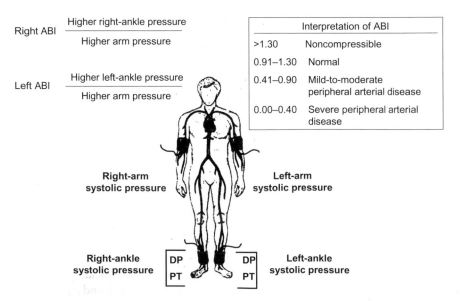

Reproduced with permission from Hiatt. NEJM. 2001

Figure 9.1 Schematic diagram showing the calculation of the ankle/brachial index.

arms and legs is a well-established noninvasive test to determine whether PAD is present and to establish a level of disease[4,5]. In order to assess flow in the limb as well, segmental limb pressures are typically measured in conjunction with segmental limb pulse volume recordings (plethysmography)[6]. Both tests are performed using pneumatic cuffs that are appropriately sized to the diameter of the limb segment under study and are properly positioned. A large limb girth as a result of extreme obesity, a large muscle mass, or edema may distort the pressure measurements. For accurate measurements, the width of the pneumatic cuff should be 20% greater than the diameter of the limb. It is common practice to evaluate the presence of arterial blood pressure in the limb distal to the cuff with an appropriate sensor (Doppler probe) prior to the measurement of pulse volume recordings.

The patient is placed in the supine position for at least 10 min prior to the measurement of the limb pressures (Figure 9.2). There are several commercially available devices that have pneumatic cuffs with automatic inflation capability. A continuous wave (CW) Doppler instrument with a transducer frequency of 4–8 MHz is the preferred instrumentation to "listen for" the arterial pulsation. The pneumatic cuff is initially inflated quickly to a suprasystolic value. The cuff is then slowly deflated until a Doppler signal returns. The cuff pressure at which the flow signal resumes is taken to be the systolic pressure in the arterial segment beneath the cuff. For example, if the cuff is on the high thigh and the sensor is in the popliteal fossa, the measured pressure is reflective of the proximal superficial femoral and profunda femoris arteries, as well as any collateral arteries, but not the popliteal artery. Although published studies have indicated that the measured pressure is slightly more accurate when the flow sensor is positioned in close proximity to the cuff, most laboratories, for convenience, use the Doppler signal from a vessel at the ankle for all limb measurements[7].

Many laboratories use a four-cuff method with the cuffs positioned as follows: (i) at the high thigh with the upper edge of the cuff positioned at the proximal portion of the inner thigh; (ii) at the low thigh above the patella; (iii) at the calf below the tibial tubercle; and (iv) at the ankle above the malleoli. An alternative method involves the use of only three cuffs with a single, relatively wide

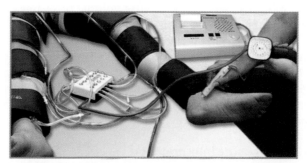

Figure 9.2 A patient undergoing segmental pressure and pulse volume recording testing using four pneumatic cuffs.

cuff at the mid-thigh. Typically, the foot pressure is measured by insonating the posterior tibial and dorsalis pedis arteries at the ankle level, thus generating two pressure numbers. Single pressure measurements are made for the calf as well as the high-thigh level and low-thigh level regardless of the tibial artery signal selected as the flow indicator. The ankle pressures are used to calculate the ABI for each extremity as noted above.

The lower extremity pressure evaluation should begin at the ankle level with a systematic search for arterial signals at ascending levels. Patients who are found to have a normal ABI are unlikely to have more proximal disease, and an exercise treadmill or reactive hyperemia test will be necessary to uncover sub-critical stenosis. If the ABI is normal and the symptoms are present in the digits of the feet, the toes should be evaluated for the presence of pedal or digital artery obstruction.

Pulse volume plethysmography technique

Plethysmography, derived from the Greek "plethysmos" meaning "increase," is used to describe the change in the volume of a limb occurring in response to blood flow into and/or out of that limb[6]. For a specific limb segment, the amplitude of the volume expansion is determined by the rate at which blood simultaneously flows in and out of the segment. In a normal cardiac cycle, blood enters the limb through the arterial system more rapidly than exiting through the venous system. This results in expansion of the limb, which is responsible for a steep, ascending systolic deflection of the pulse volume recording. After peak expansion of the limb has been achieved, blood exits more rapidly than it enters, resulting in a return to the end-diastolic or pre-expansion volume. The resulting descending deflection of the normal pulse volume is more prolonged than the ascending deflection. The pulse volume curve is analogous to the arterial pressure pulse. A cuff pressure of 65 mmHg has been found to achieve surface contact of the cuff to the skin and at the same time impart a reproducible contour characteristic of plethysmography. The signal amplitude may, however, be affected by factors such as the ventricular stroke volume, blood pressure, vascular tone, arrhythmia, and position of the limb. In addition, the amplitude is affected by exercise.

Segmental limb plethysmography (pulse volume recording) is performed using pneumatic cuffs, which are appropriately sized to the diameter of the limb segment under study and are properly positioned. Each cuff is sequentially inflated to a predetermined reference pressure (i.e. 65 mmHg). Plethysmographic waveforms are recorded for each limb segment. Of note, the cuff placement may need to be readjusted to ensure that the reference cuff pressure can be achieved within a narrow range of cuff inflation volume. Bilateral testing is considered as an integral part of each examination.

Segmental limb pressure interpretation

Systolic intravascular pressures increase slightly from the femoral to the tibial level, so that the intra-arterial measurement of pressures typically demonstrates

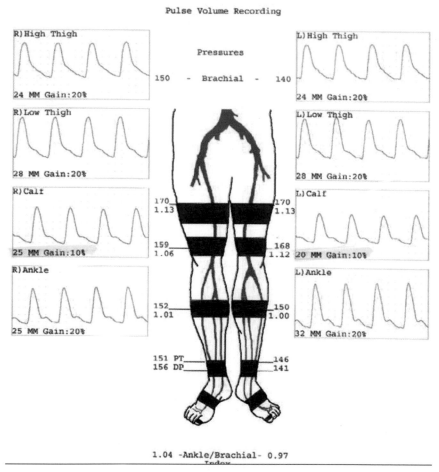

Figure 9.3 Normal segmental pressure and pulse volume recording study.

a higher pressure in the tibial artery than in the femoral artery. When the four-cuff method is used with relatively narrow cuffs, a pressure artifact is introduced into the measurement, accounting for the gradual increase in the measured pressure in ascending levels of the leg. In healthy subjects, the high thigh pressure typically exceeds the ankle pressure by approximately 30 mmHg[5]. Thus, a thigh/brachial index of 1.1 or greater is indicative of normal hemodynamics (Figure 9.3), and an index of less than 0.8 is indicative of proximal occlusion (Figure 9.4). Of note, when the high thigh pressure is low compared with the brachial artery pressure, the level of obstruction may be proximal to the cuff or beneath the cuff. Thus, the site of obstruction could be in the aorta, iliac artery, common femoral artery, profunda (deep) femoris, or proximal superficial femoral artery. When the inflow hemodynamics are abnormal bilater-

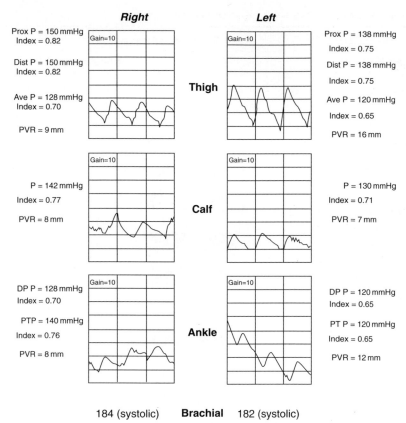

Right

Prox P = 150 mmHg
Index = 0.82

Dist P = 150 mmHg
Index = 0.82

Ave P = 128 mmHg
Index = 0.70

PVR = 9 mm

Left

Prox P = 138 mmHg
Index = 0.75

Dist P = 138 mmHg
Index = 0.75

Ave P = 120 mmHg
Index = 0.65

PVR = 16 mm

Thigh

P = 142 mmHg
Index = 0.77
PVR = 8 mm

Calf

P = 130 mmHg
Index = 0.71
PVR = 7 mm

DP P = 128 mmHg
Index = 0.70
PTP = 140 mmHg
Index = 0.76
PVR = 8 mm

Ankle

DP P = 120 mmHg
Index = 0.65
PT P = 120 mmHg
Index = 0.65
PVR = 12 mm

184 (systolic)   **Brachial**   182 (systolic)

Figure 9.4 An elderly patient with a right and left thigh/brachial index of < 0.8 indicating arterial occlusion. This patient was found to have an occluded aorta with collateral vessels seen on contrast aortography.

ally, the site of obstruction is the aorto-iliac region. However, if the decrease in pressures is unilateral, only an ipsilateral iliac or common femoral artery stenosis is inferred, and an abnormality of the aortic segment should not be included in the interpretation.

The segmental limb pressures are compared with adjacent ipsilateral segments, with the contralateral paired segment, and with the greater of the two brachial systolic pressures (Table 9.1). A 20 mmHg or greater decrease in pressures is considered to be significant if such a gradient is present either between segments along the same leg or when compared with the same level of the opposite leg[8]. A pressure gradient across the thigh of > 30 mmHg is considered to be diagnostic for superficial femoral, popliteal, and infra-popliteal artery disease. Toe pressures may also be measured and the toe pressure index (TPI) can be generated. A TPI $\geq$ 80% of the brachial or 60% of the ankle systolic pressure is considered to be normal.

Table 9.1 Criteria for abnormal segmental pressure study.

Level of disease	Findings
Aorto-iliac	High thigh/brachial index < 1.1 bilaterally
Iliac	High thigh/brachial index < 1.1 unilaterally
Superficial femoral artery (SFA) disease*	Gradient between high and low thigh cuffs
Distal SFA/popliteal*	Gradient between thigh and calf cuffs
Infra-popliteal*	Gradient between calf and ankle cuffs

*Pressure gradient between 20 and 30 mmHg is borderline, ≥ 30 mmHg is abnormal.
This is an indirect examination on which the anatomic location is inferred based on hemodynamic findings. Multiple vessels located at or above the level of the pneumatic cuff may not be separated.

Pulse volume plethysmography interpretation

Segmental limb plethysmographic waveform analysis is based on the evaluation of the signal amplitude and waveform shape. Standardized criteria relating waveform changes to anatomic site and hemodynamic severity of disease are utilized in the diagnostic interpretation. Pulse volume recordings are typically performed by injecting a standard volume of air into pneumatic cuffs. Older vintage machines, such as Life Sciences, were adjusted for the amount of air in the cuff so that a precise comparison could be made between the legs or at various levels along the extremities. Many newer machines, however, do not calibrate the amount of air in the cuff; thus, caution is advised in interpreting the amplitude of the pulse volume recording in comparison with the other extremity or at various levels. The volume of air injected into the cuff is sufficient to occlude the venous circulation, but does not occlude the arterial circulation.

Volume changes in the limb segment below the cuff are translated into a pulsatile pressure, which is detected by a transducer and then displayed by a pressure pulse contour. A normal pulse volume recording, similar to the arterial waveform, is composed of a systolic upstroke with a sharp systolic peak followed by a downstroke that contains a prominent dicrotic notch. If a hemodynamically significant stenosis is present, dissipation of energy occurs as a result of arterial narrowing, and this is reflected in a change in the pulse volume recording contour indicating a proximal arterial obstruction. The amount of variation in the pulse volume recording contour is reflective of disease severity (Figure 9.5). For example, mild disease is characterized by the absence of a dicrotic notch, whereas, with moderate disease, the upstroke and downstroke become equal. Severe disease is characterized by a flat or significantly blunted waveform. An advantage of using pulse volume recording amplitudes is that they are valid when examining calcified vessels, as the test does not rely on occlusion of the calcified artery.

Limitations

The evaluation of segmental pressures and volume plethysmography represents an indirect examination on which the anatomic location of lesions is inferred based on hemodynamic findings. Multiple vessels located at or above the

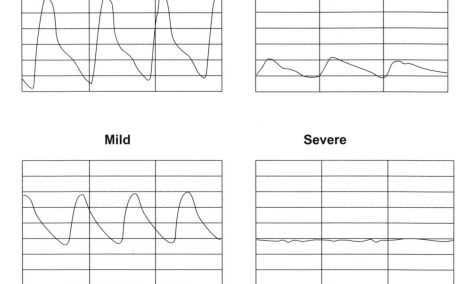

Figure 9.5 Examples of pulse volume recordings demonstrating mild, moderate, and severe waveforms.

level of the pneumatic cuff may not be separated. For example, a decreased thigh pressure may be caused by obstruction of the aorto-iliac segment or common femoral artery, or combined superficial femoral artery and profundus femoris artery disease. In addition, these physiologic tests do not discriminate between stenosis and occlusion of the arterial segment, nor can they determine the length of arterial lesions.

Exercise testing for peripheral arterial disease

Indications for treadmill testing
PAD may be revealed by measurement of the lower extremity pressures after exercise[9,10]. Indications for stress testing of the lower extremities include: normal resting lower extremity arterial segmental limb pressures and pulse volume recordings in the context of a history suggestive of intermittent claudication; resting lower extremity segmental limb pressures and pulse volume recording amplitudes mildly abnormal at rest (i.e. ABI > 0.80 but < 0.96); and a patient with a history of intermittent claudication.

Contraindications to treadmill testing
Contraindications to exercise treadmill testing of the lower extremities include

rest pain, tissue loss, necrosis or ulceration of the lower extremities, noncompressible vessels on a resting study, acute deep venous thrombosis, shortness of breath at rest or with minimal exertion, uncontrolled angina, or a physical disability which limits a patient's ability to ambulate on a treadmill (i.e. balance or gait disturbances).

Exercise treadmill technique

Patients are instructed to fast for 12 h prior to the treadmill test. Prior to walking on the treadmill, patients are given detailed instructions together with a demonstration. These include alerting the technician with regard to the development of pain, not leaning onto the handrails, and reporting any chest discomfort or dyspnea that may develop. The standard treadmill protocol uses a speed of two miles per hour and a 12% grade. The duration of the test is typically 5 min, or shorter if the patient cannot continue due to claudication symptoms. The exercise treadmill study is stopped immediately if the patient develops chest pain or dyspnea, or if other symptoms (such as dizziness) impair the patient's ability to continue. The treadmill test is discontinued after the patient has completed 5 min of exercise, or if symptoms force the patient to stop.

After the treadmill has stopped, the patient is immediately returned to the supine position. The ankle pressures are obtained initially, starting with the symptomatic leg. The ankle pressures are recorded every minute for 5 min. Some laboratories evaluate the ankle pressures for up to 10 min. The pressure measurement routine is stopped earlier if the pressure returns to baseline. Of note, the brachial/systolic pressure should be recorded immediately at the first set of ankle pressures and at the end of the post-exercise ankle pressures. If available, a second technologist should take the brachial pressures so as not to delay the measurement of the ankle pressures. The data recorded from the treadmill procedure should include the measured ankle pressures, the length of time the patient was able to walk, the time required for the pressure to return to baseline, the nature and location of the patient's symptoms, and the reason for discontinuing the test.

Plantar flexion exercise

An alternative method for stress testing for patients unable to walk is active pedal plantar flexion. This exercise test involves the patient standing on a foot stool and performing repetitive toe raises to exercise the calf muscles. The patient is instructed to stand initially with finger support for balance, using the rail for balance only. The patient should extend the feet fully and return to the baseline stance, performing up to 50 repetitions, or until he or she is unable to continue. The number of "toe-ups" completed at the onset of discomfort in the calves should be recorded. In addition, the number of repetitions performed should be recorded. After completing the exercise regimen, the patient should be rapidly returned to the supine position. The ankle pressure should be measured immediately, as well as at 1–2 min intervals after the cessation of exercise for 10 min, or until the baseline resting pressure is reached. The brachial systolic pressure should be recorded immediately after the first set of ankle pressures and at the end of the post-exercise ankle pressures. If available, a second technologist should measure the brachial pressure so as not to delay the measurement of the ankle pressures.

Reference list

1 Hirsch AT, Criqui MH, Treat-Jacobson D, *et al*. Peripheral arterial disease detection, awareness, and treatment in primary care. J Am Med Assoc 2001; 286(11):1317–1324.

2 Newman AB, Sutton-Tyrrell K, Vogt MT, Kuller LH. Morbidity and mortality in hypertensive adults with a low ankle/arm blood pressure index. J Am Med Assoc 1993; 270:487–489.

3 Resnick HE, Lindsay RS, McDermott MM, *et al*. Relationship of high and low ankle brachial index to all-cause and cardiovascular disease mortality: the Strong Heart Study. Circulation 2004; 109(6):733–739.

4 Winsor T. Instrumental methods for studying the peripheral arterial circulation. Cardiovasc Clin 1971; 3(1):17–35.

5 Heintz SE, Bone GE, Slaymaker EE, Hayes AC, Barnes RW. Value of arterial pressure measurements in the proximal and distal part of the thigh in arterial occlusive disease. Surg Gynecol Obstet 1978; 146:337–343.

6 Darling RC, Raines JK, Brener BJ, Austen WG. Quantitative segmental pulse volume recorder: a clinical tool. Surgery 1972; 72:873–887.

7 Franzeck UK, Bernstein EF, Fronek A. The effect of sensing site on the limb segmental blood pressure determination. Arch Surg 1981; 116(7):912–916.

8 Fronek A, Johansen KH, Dilley RB, Bernstein EF. Noninvasive physiologic tests in the diagnosis and characterization of peripheral arterial occlusive disease. Am J Surg 1973; 126(2):205–214.

9 Carter SA. Clinical measurement of systolic pressures in limbs with arterial occlusive disease. J Am Med Assoc 1969; 207(10):1869–1874.

10 Carter SA. Response of ankle systolic pressure to leg exercise in mild or questionable arterial disease. N Engl J Med 1972; 287(12):578–582.

10 Peripheral Arterial Ultrasonography

Marie Gerhard-Herman and Emile R. Mohler III

Duplex ultrasound

Duplex ultrasound is easily applied to the evaluation of peripheral arteries[1]. Peripheral arterial ultrasound is not routinely used as a screening test for the diagnosis of peripheral arterial disease (PAD), but rather is performed to localize and grade the severity of arterial stenosis in patients with exercise-associated limb discomfort or following peripheral arterial revascularization. Segmental pressure measurements and pulse volume recordings (see Chapter 9) are commonly used in vascular laboratories as the initial evaluation for PAD, but some laboratories begin with an assessment of the ankle/brachial index and, if abnormal, proceed directly to arterial duplex ultrasound. Duplex ultrasound allows for the determination of the exact site of the disease and for the discrimination between stenosis and occlusion, and identifies aneurysmal disease. In addition, peripheral arterial ultrasound is versatile and mobile, as it can be performed urgently at the bedside in the setting of an acutely ischemic limb. This chapter focuses on lower extremity arterial ultrasound.

Anatomy of the lower extremity arteries

The distal aorta bifurcates into the right and left common iliac arteries at the level of the umbilicus (Figure 10.1). The common iliac artery divides into the internal iliac and external iliac arteries at the beginning of the sacral spine. The internal iliac artery courses medially. The larger external iliac artery becomes the common femoral artery as it passes under the inguinal ligament. The main branches of the external iliac artery are the inferior epigastric and deep circumflex arteries that provide blood supply to the abdominal muscles. The common femoral artery branches into the superficial and deep femoral (profunda femoris) arteries. The superficial femoral artery becomes the popliteal artery as it passes through the adductor canal proximal to the knee joint.

The popliteal artery divides in the proximal calf into the tibioperoneal trunk and the anterior tibial artery. The anterior tibial artery courses anterolaterally and becomes the dorsalis pedis artery as it crosses the ankle onto the dorsum of the foot. The tibioperoneal trunk divides soon after its origin into the peroneal

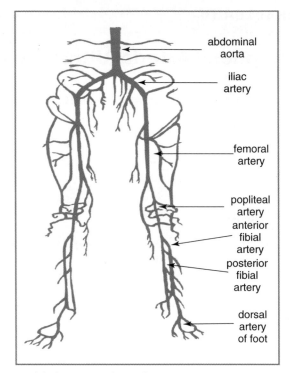

abdominal
aorta

iliac
artery

femoral
artery

popliteal
artery

anterior
fibial
artery

posterior
fibial
artery

dorsal
artery
of foot

Figure 10.1 Anatomy of the lower extremity arteries.

and posterior tibial arteries. The posterior tibial artery continues in a posterior and medial direction, dividing into medial and lateral plantar arteries when it enters the foot. The dorsalis pedis artery gives rise to the deep plantar artery that joins the lateral plantar artery to form the plantar arch. The peroneal artery courses laterally and provides peroneal perforators which supply blood to the calf musculature.

Duplex examination of the native arteries

The lower extremity arteries are evaluated using gray scale images, color Doppler, and spectral Doppler analysis[2]. Color Doppler and transverse imaging are utilized to identify the vessels (Figure 10.2). Bowel gas can obscure the visualization of the iliac arteries. It is therefore optimal to evaluate the iliac arteries in a fasting patient. Significant abdominal adiposity may also obscure the identification of these vessels. The probe is turned longitudinally to perform the Doppler evaluation. Color Doppler identifies laminar flow in normal arteries, while turbulence and aliasing are evident in stenotic arteries. The sample volume must be as small as possible and in the center stream of the arterial flow in order to avoid spectral broadening. It may be advantageous to increase the sample volume at the point of an occlusion or stenosis. The Doppler gain should be

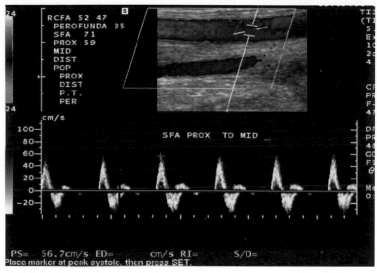

Figure 10.2 Color Doppler ultrasound image with spectral Doppler showing a normal superficial femoral artery.

kept just below the threshold of background noise, and a low wall filter (50 Hz) is advised.

The spectral Doppler evaluation is performed with the Doppler sample cursor parallel to the inner wall of the artery and forming a 60° angle with the insonation beam. The "heel–toe" technique with the transducer optimizes the angles and minimizes "steering" in different directions. The sites at which the waveforms should be recorded are the common iliac, external iliac, common femoral, profunda femoris, superficial femoral, and popliteal arteries. The superficial femoral artery waveform should be recorded in the proximal, mid- and distal portions, with special attention paid to the adductor canal.

A 3–5 MHz probe is used to visualize the common iliac arteries at the level of the umbilicus. The distal external iliac and common femoral arteries can typically be evaluated with a 5.0 MHz probe. Initially, the transverse view is used to identify the common femoral artery and origins of the superficial femoral artery and profunda femoris artery. The transducer is rotated to obtain a long-axis view of the common femoral artery. Gray scale imaging is performed from the proximal to distal thigh to evaluate the course of the superficial femoral artery and to determine the presence of plaque and other luminal abnormalities. Color and spectral Doppler sampling is then performed throughout the femoral artery from the medial approach. Aliasing, turbulence, and elevation of the systolic velocities are all signs of stenosis[3,4]. Of note, color flow Doppler, similar to spectral Doppler, depends on the angle between the ultrasound beam and the direction of blood flow, and will only be accurate if this angle is set and remains constant along the length of a vessel. Thus, color differences in a vessel that is not straight may represent either true velocity changes or a variation in the frequency shift resulting from changes in the Doppler angle (see Chapter 2).

The patient lifts the leg, rolls onto the side, or changes to the prone position in order to evaluate the popliteal artery from a posterior approach. Higher frequency probes are used at the level of the popliteal artery and distally. The leg is rotated outwards in order to evaluate the peroneal and posterior tibial arteries from a medial approach. Some sonographers scan from the popliteal space down the leg and others begin at the ankle and scan proximally. The anterior tibial artery is examined using an anterolateral approach. The tibial and peroneal arteries each lie between two veins. A single vein is evident paired with each popliteal, femoral, and iliac artery. The veins are larger in caliber compared with the arteries and compress with relatively less pressure. However, veins may contract due to resolving thrombus and may become similar in caliber or even smaller than arteries.

Definition of peripheral arterial stenosis

The spectral Doppler waveform is used to quantify stenosis in the peripheral arteries and is based on the principle that the velocity of blood flow increases through a narrow region in the bloodstream. One schema utilizes the analysis of the waveform characteristics of spectral broadening and peak systolic velocity (Table 10.1)[5]. The sensitivity of duplex ultrasound for the detection of a stenosis or occlusion is approximately 88–95%, with a specificity of 95–99% and an accuracy of 93%[3,6]. The normal arterial waveform from the level of the abdominal aorta to the tibial arteries is triphasic with a clear window below the systolic peak. A gradual decrease in the peak systolic velocity occurs from the distal aorta throughout the distal arterial segments. The normal value of the peak sys-

Table 10.1 Criteria for the classification of peripheral artery lesions based on duplex scanning with spectral waveform analysis.

Lesion	Criteria
Normal	Triphasic waveform, no spectral broadening
20–49% diameter reduction	Triphasic waveform usually maintained, although reverse flow component may be diminished; spectral broadening is prominent with filling in of the clear area under the systolic peak; peak systolic velocity is increased from 30% to 100% relative to the adjacent proximal segment; proximal and distal waveforms remain normal
50–99% diameter reduction	Monophasic waveform with loss of the reverse flow component and forward flow throughout the cardiac cycle; extensive spectral broadening; peak systolic velocity is increased > 100% relative to the adjacent proximal segment; distal waveform is monophasic with reduced systolic velocity
Occlusion	No flow detected within the imaged arterial segment; pre-occlusive "thump" may be heard just proximal to the site of occlusion; distal waveforms are monophasic with reduced systolic velocities

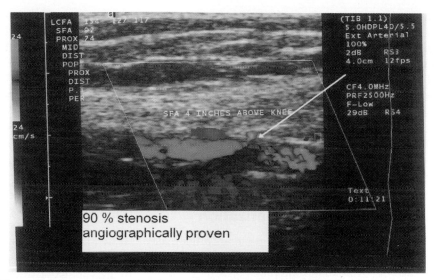

Figure 10.3 Color Doppler tracing of a superficial artery showing a stenosis of approximately 90%.

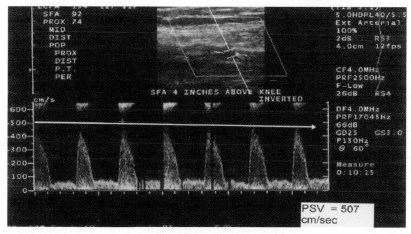

Figure 10.4 Spectral Doppler tracing showing quadrupled systolic velocity compared with the proximal normal segment, spectral broadening, and loss of reverse flow, consistent with > 75% stenosis.

tolic velocity in the aorta is $100\ \text{cm s}^{-1}$ and decreases to approximately $70\ \text{cm s}^{-1}$ in the popliteal artery (Figure 10.3).

There is no stenosis in the absence of spectral broadening or an increase in peak systolic velocity with sequential (proximal to distal) Doppler sampling. An increase, but not doubling, of the peak systolic velocity, accompanied by spectral broadening, indicates 1–49% stenosis. Doubling of the peak systolic velocity in sequential samples with marked spectral broadening and loss of reverse flow indicates 50–99% stenosis (Figure 10.4). A reduction in arterial diameter of 50% or greater commonly results in a pressure gradient with exertion and the development of claudication symptoms. When the peak systolic velocity quadruples from one segment to the next, greater than 75% stenosis or lumen diameter reduction is present. As the degree of stenosis increases, the spectral waveform changes progressively from normal triphasic flow to monophasic flow in severe stenosis. Ratios of the peak systolic velocities correlate more strongly with stenosis than do mean ratios of the systolic velocities[3].

Ultrasound evaluation after percutaneous revascularization

The long-term patency of percutaneous angioplasty and stenting in the lower extremities varies between clinical trials and lies in the range 50–85%[7–9]. Duplex ultrasound evaluation should be performed shortly after percutaneous revascularization in order to document the level of success and to identify individuals who may need re-intervention. Follow-up ultrasound evaluation should also be performed annually or if leg symptoms suggestive of ischemia occur.

The examination post-revascularization must include the native artery proximal and distal to the site of revascularization[10]. The entire length of the artery under study is first evaluated with transverse and longitudinal color Doppler. The spectral Doppler sample volume is then "marched" through the artery from the proximal native artery to the distal native artery[11]. The pulsed wave sample cursor is placed parallel to the inner wall and at an angle of 60° with respect to the insonation beam. Stenosis is evaluated in a manner similar to that utilized in native arteries described above. A peak systolic velocity ratio of two indicates stenosis greater than 50%[3]. The fundamental criteria of duplex evaluation following percutaneous revascularization include: (i) peak systolic velocities of > 180 cm s^{-1} and peak systolic velocity ratios of more than two are significant; and (ii) changes in waveform shape and velocity measurements on serial examinations.

Ultrasound evaluation after surgical revascularization

It is estimated that 20–30% of patients undergoing a surgical bypass graft revascularization will develop graft thrombosis as a result of graft failure. Early detection of a graft stenosis, with subsequent repair, results in improved long-term patency when compared with the occurrence of thrombosis requiring emergency graft thrombectomy and repair. Thus, scheduled graft surveillance is crucial in preserving bypass patency. Graft surveillance after infra-inguinal bypass begins in the operating room using ultrasound to verify that the arterial bypass has no stenosis and has sufficient arterial blood flow for patency (Table 10.2). A complete graft ultrasound evaluation, usually accompanied by ankle/brachial

Table 10.2 Bypass graft abnormalities at the time of operation.

Vein conduit stenosis and fibrosis
Hemodynamic stenosis from small caliber conduit
Anastomotic stenosis
Inadequate vein valve lysis
Inflow and outflow artery obstruction or stenosis
Arterial clamp injury
Low graft flow velocity due to diseased runoff arteries

Table 10.3 Risk stratification for graft thrombosis based on surveillance data.

Category*	High-velocity criteria	Low-velocity criteria	ΔABI
I (highest risk)	$PSV > 300$ cm s^{-1} or Vr > 3.5 and	$GFV < 45$ cm s^{-1}	or > 0.15
II (high risk)	$PSV > 300$ cm s^{-1} or Vr > 3.5 and	$GFV > 45$ cm s^{-1}	and < 0.15
III (intermediate risk)	$180 < PSV > 300$ cm s^{-1} or Vr > 2.0 and	$GFV > 45$ cm s^{-1}	and < 0.15
IV (low risk)	$PSV < 180$ cm s^{-1} and Vr < 2.0 and	$GFV > 45$ cm s^{-1}	and < 0.15

*Category I: patients are hospitalized and anticoagulated; lesions are repaired promptly. Category II: lesions are repaired electively (within 2 weeks). Category III: lesions are closely observed with serial duplex examination and are repaired only if they progress. Category IV: lesions are at low risk (we have observed few failures in this group).
ABI = Doppler-derived ankle/brachial index; GFV = graft flow velocity (global or distal); PSV – duplex-derived peak systolic velocity at site of flow disturbance; Vr = velocity ratio of stenosis to more proximal graft segment of same caliber. (Adapted with permission from Bandyk DF. Infrainguinal vein bypass graft surveillance: how to do it, when to intervene, and is it cost-effective? J Am Coll Surg 2002; 194(1 Suppl.):S40–S52.)

index and ankle pulse volume recordings, should be performed prior to discharge or within 7 days after surgery. Subsequent ultrasound studies should occur at 1 month, followed by 3 month intervals for the first year[12]. If the graft remains normal after the first year, a follow-up study is recommended every 6 months. However, grafts with an abnormal duplex ultrasound shortly after surgery require careful and frequent duplex ultrasound surveillance.

The bypass graft study involves the evaluation of the proximal native artery, proximal anastomosis, entire graft conduit, distal anastomosis, and distal outflow artery[12]. The examination technique and interpretation of the findings are identical for native artery evaluation pre- and post-angioplasty. In contrast, arterial bypass grafts present with distinct findings, such as abrupt changes in diameter secondary to mismatch between the graft and native vessel or between segments of graft constructed from different veins[13]. The phenomenon of mismatch is most evident at the distal anastomosis. In this setting, a tripling in the peak systolic velocity is needed to diagnose significant stenosis of the distal anastomosis. In addition, bypass grafts have an increased likelihood of thrombosis when there is low flow (Table 10.3). Peak systolic velocities of less than 40 cm s^{-1} are consistent with an impending graft thrombosis[14]. The peak systolic velocity and peak systolic velocity ratios are used to categorize bypass graft stenosis[12].

Findings other than stenosis

Popliteal, superficial femoral, and iliac artery aneurysms can be identified on duplex ultrasound. Aneurysm is diagnosed when the diameter of the vessel doubles from one segment to the next. Thrombus is frequently detected lining the aneurysm cavity. Thrombus can progress to obliterate the arterial lumen. Thrombus can also embolize distally, resulting in arterial occlusion characterized by an abrupt cut-off in arterial flow. Adventitial cysts are also found in the wall of the popliteal artery.

Calf pain with activity and relieved by rest is also caused by entrapment of the popliteal artery by the medial head of the gastrocnemius muscle (Figure 10.5). The distal popliteal artery can be evaluated during gastrocnemius flexion maneuvers[15,16]. An increase in peak systolic velocity of at least 50% during maneuvers is consistent with the diagnosis of popliteal entrapment. The diagnosis of early compartment syndrome, causing calf pain with activity, cannot be made with ultrasound.

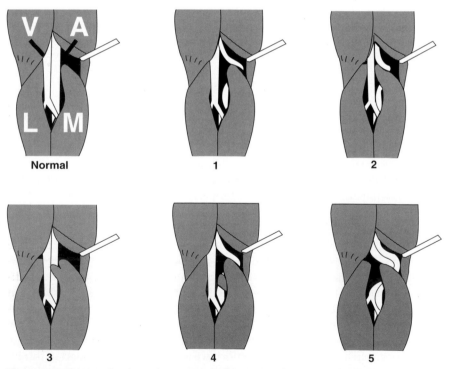

Figure 10.5 Diagram showing various anatomic abnormalities that may result in popliteal entrapment.

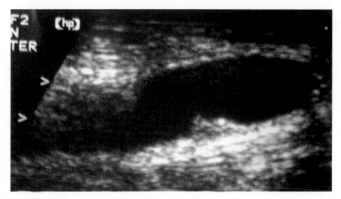

Figure 10.6 Ultrasound image of a patient with a Baker's cyst in the popliteal fossa.

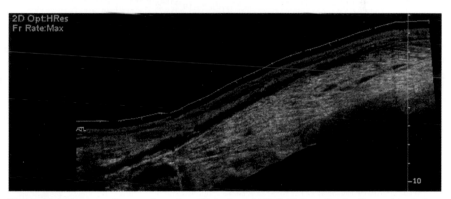

Figure 10.7 Ultrasound image of a ruptured Baker's cyst with fluid dissecting the tissue plane in the popliteal fossa.

Other findings, such as adventitial cyst disease or popliteal (Baker's) cyst, may be noted in the popliteal space on ultrasound imaging. Adventitial cyst disease of the popliteal artery may be seen in a patient, usually male and less than 50 years of age, with sudden onset of claudication symptoms, but without the risk factors commonly associated with claudication. Multilobulated cysts are seen on ultrasound arising from the wall of the artery. The arterial lumen and blood flow are preserved. An angiogram may show a focal, smooth tapered stenosis at the level of the femoral condyles. A Baker's cyst appears as a discrete hypoechoic structure in the popliteal fossa (Figure 10.6) as a result of posterior herniation of the synovium through the knee joint capsule, or distension of the gastrocnemius semimembranous bursa that fills through a normal communication with the knee joint. If the Baker's cyst has ruptured, there is no discrete cystic structure and fluid dissects into the calf, but usually superficial to the popliteal artery (Figure 10.7).

Reference list

1 Strandness DE Jr, Schultz RD, Sumner DS, Rushmer RF. Ultrasonic flow detection. A useful technique in the evaluation of peripheral vascular disease. Am J Surg 1967; 113(3):311–320.

2 Jager KA, Phillips DJ, Martin RL, *et al*. Noninvasive mapping of lower limb arterial lesions. Ultrasound Med Biol 1985; 11(3):515–521.

3 Polak J. Determinations of the extent of lower extremity peripheral arterial disease with color-assisted duplex sonography: comparison with angiography. Am J Roentgenol 1990; 155:1085–1089.

4 Pellerito J. Color persistence: indicator of hemodynamically significant peripheral arterial stenosis. Radiology 1991; 181:89.

5 Cossman DV, Ellison JE, Wagner WH, *et al*. Comparison of contrast arteriography to arterial mapping with color-flow duplex imaging in the lower extremities. J Vasc Surg 1989; 10(5):522–528.

6 Ranke C, Creutzig A, Alexander K. Duplex scanning of the peripheral arteries: correlation of the peak velocity ratio with angiographic diameter reduction. Ultrasound Med Biol 1992; 18:433–440.

7 Matsi PJ, Manninen HI, Soder HK, Mustonen P, Kouri J. Percutaneous transluminal angioplasty in femoral artery occlusions: primary and long-term results in 107 claudicant patients using femoral and popliteal catheterization techniques. Clin Radiol 1995; 50(4):237–244.

8 Cejna M, Thurnher S, Illiasch H, *et al*. PTA versus Palmaz stent placement in femoropopliteal artery obstructions: a multicenter prospective randomized study. J Vasc Intervent Radiol 2001; 12(1):23–31.

9 Soder HK, Manninen HI, Rasanen HT, Kaukanen E, Jaakkola P, Matsi PJ. Failure of prolonged dilation to improve long-term patency of femoropopliteal artery angioplasty: results of a prospective trial. J Vasc Intervent Radiol 2002; 13(4):361–369.

10 Roth SM, Bandyk DF. Duplex imaging of lower extremity bypasses, angioplasties, and stents. Semin Vasc Surg 1999; 12(4):275–284.

11 Ahn SS, Rutherford RB, Becker GJ, *et al*. Reporting standards for lower extremity arterial endovascular procedures. Society for Vascular Surgery/International Society for Cardio-vascular Surgery. J Vasc Surg 1993; 17(6):1103–1107.

12 Bandyk DF. Infrainguinal vein bypass graft surveillance: how to do it, when to intervene, and is it cost-effective? J Am Coll Surg 2002; 194(1 Suppl.):S40–S52.

13 Armstrong PA, Bandyk DF, Wilson JS, Shames ML, Johnson BL, Back MR. Optimizing infrainguinal arm vein bypass patency with duplex ultrasound surveillance and endovas-cular therapy. J Vasc Surg 2004; 40(4):724–730.

14 Bandyk DF, Cato RF, Towne JB. A low flow velocity predicts failure of femoropopliteal and femorotibial bypass grafts. Surgery 1985; 98(4):799–809.

15 Miles S, Roediger W, Cooke P, Mieny CJ. Doppler ultrasound in the diagnosis of the popliteal artery entrapment syndrome. Br J Surg 1977; 64(12):883–884.

16 Chernoff DM, Walker AT, Khorasani R, Polak JF, Jolesz FA. Asymptomatic functional popliteal artery entrapment: demonstration at MR imaging. Radiology 1995; 195(1): 176–180.

11 | Thoracic Outlet Evaluation

Edward Y. Woo, Julia T. Davis and Jeffrey P. Carpenter

Introduction

Thoracic outlet syndrome (TOS) comprises nerve, artery, or vein compression as it traverses the thoracic outlet. This can be asymptomatic or can lead to symptoms in the upper extremities. Neurogenic TOS is the most common. However, compression of the artery or vein is also important. History and physical examination are important for the diagnosis. Moreover, multiple studies are useful for confirming the diagnosis. It is imperative to rule out other diseases that may present in a similar manner. Treatment of TOS is tailored to the type and degree of disease.

Anatomy

The thoracic outlet is defined by the space formed from the vertebral column, sternum, and first rib. The anterior and middle scalene muscles attach to the first rib anteromedially and medially, respectively. This space allows for the course of the subclavian artery and brachial plexus (Figure 11.1). Furthermore, the subclavian vein travels anterior to the anterior scalene. This space is somewhat constrained and anomalies in this area can lead to the development of TOS. For example, cervical ribs or abnormalities of the scalene muscles can cause compressive symptoms.

Thoracic outlet syndrome

Neurogenic

The brachial plexus comprises spinal nerves C5 to T1. These nerves travel between the anterior and middle scalene muscles. There are many postulated factors that can result in compression of these nerves (Figure 11.2). Cervical ribs, which are rare, course through the middle scalene muscle and can impinge upon the nerves. Variations in the normal anatomy of the scalene muscles can also lead to nerve entrapment (Figure 11.2). For example, splitting of the anterior scalene muscle around the nerve or fibrous extensions from either the anterior or middle scalene can lead to compression. Neurogenic TOS usually results from neck trauma superimposed on one of the above or other predisposing fac-

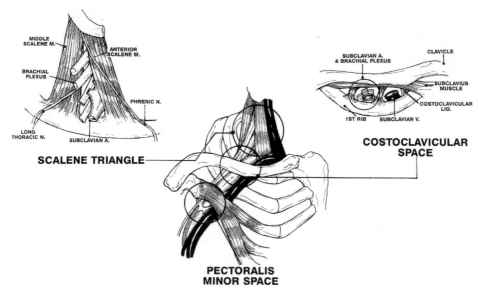

Figure 11.1 Multiple views are shown demonstrating the normal course of the neurovascular bundle through the thoracic outlet. Reprinted from Rutherford RB (ed.) *Vascular Surgery*, Sanders R, Cooper M, Hammond S, Weinstein S, Neurogenic thoracic outlet syndrome, page 1185, Copyright 2000, with permission from Elsevier.

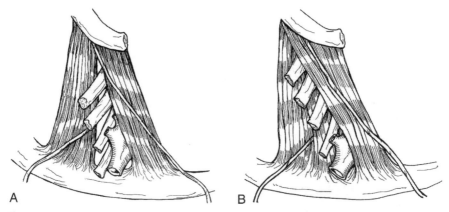

Figure 11.2 Note the comparison between a normal and abnormal interscalene space. The brachial plexus is entrapped by the scalene muscles. Reprinted from Rutherford RB (ed.) *Vascular Surgery*, Sanders R, Cooper M, Hammond S, Weinstein S, Neurogenic thoracic outlet syndrome, page 1187, Copyright 2000, with permission from Elsevier.

tors. Symptoms often include pain or aching, paresthesia, numbness, and weakness of the affected extremity. Symptoms are most commonly present along the ulnar distribution.

The diagnosis of neurogenic TOS ultimately depends on the clinical findings. Classic findings on history and physical examination are important. Objective studies can then confirm the disease process. The treatment of TOS begins with physical therapy and rehabilitation. Neck stretching, abdominal breathing, and postural exercises are the mainstay[1]. These maneuvers are meant to relax the neck muscles. Medications for pain relief and anxiety can be added. Avoidance of activities that worsen the symptoms should be advised. If physical therapy is unsuccessful, surgery may be warranted.

The ultimate goal of surgery is to relieve all compression of the nerves in the thoracic outlet. Two main approaches have evolved. Scalenectomy, i.e. resection of the anterior and middle scalene muscles, is performed under the assumption that variations in muscle anatomy are responsible. On surgery, fibrous bands impinging on the nerves or aberrant muscle fibers entrapping the nerves may be found. The release of these bands and fibers decompresses the nerve bundle as it traverses the thoracic outlet. The other approach is rib resection. If a cervical rib is present, it can be resected through a supraclavicular approach. More importantly, decompression can also be achieved by removing the first rib, and thus widening the thoracic outlet. This can be performed via a transaxillary, supraclavicular, or infraclavicular approach.

At times, both scalenectomy and rib resection may be warranted. In either event, care must be taken in dissection around this area. The brachial plexus, thoracodorsal nerve, long thoracic nerve, phrenic nerve, thoracic duct, subclavian artery, and subclavian vein are in the immediate vicinity. Furthermore, inadvertent injury to the pleura and lung must be avoided.

The success of the procedure is variable, and is usually defined by at least partial relief of the symptoms. It is uncommon for all of the symptoms to be resolved. As there is no standard by which to measure success, subjective evaluation by the patient is used. Surgery often provides sufficient relief to allow a return to work, as well as a significant improvement in lifestyle.

Arterial

TOS secondary to arterial lesions is much less common than neurogenic TOS. It is usually a result of compression of the artery as it exits the thoracic outlet. Presentation occurs in an older age group. Compression is most often due to bony abnormalities, including cervical ribs or variations of the first rib. Only rarely do fibrous bands or scalene muscle aberrations lead to arterial TOS. The natural course of this pathologic process involves progressive narrowing and stenosis of the artery. In time, these lesions become quite significant and difficult to treat. Furthermore, patients can develop post-stenotic aneurysmal dilation of the subclavian artery. Thromboembolic disease with resultant extremity ischemia is the main complication. It is unusual for the stenosis or even occlusion to cause significant arm ischemia secondary to the rich collateral supply through the shoulder girdle. However, a flow-limiting lesion in combination with poor distal runoff secondary to thromboembolic disease can lead to significant ischemia.

The presentation of arterial TOS can be similar to that of its neurogenic counterpart. Other manifestations can include thromboembolic phenomena and digital ischemia, or a pulsatile aneurysm in the upper thorax. Often, these lesions can be found incidentally. Treatment of arterial TOS involves two components. First, decompression of the thoracic outlet needs to be accomplished. Resection of a cervical rib or resection of the first rib is usually all that is necessary. This can usually be accomplished through a supraclavicular or transaxillary approach. Treatment of the arterial lesion is the other component. Stenotic lesions can be bypassed if necessary. However, these lesions may be amenable to endovascular angioplasty and stenting. Aneurysms of the subclavian artery can also be treated with a traditional open procedure, such as aneurysmorraphy. At the same time, placement of a covered stent may successfully exclude the aneurysm[2]. Finally, distal ischemia may also need to be addressed. Thromboembolectomy or distal bypass may be warranted to alleviate the ischemia.

Venous

Primary thrombosis of the subclavian and axillary veins has been termed "Paget–Schroetter" disease. Venous TOS or "effort thrombosis" must be distinguished from other causes of central venous thrombosis, such as indwelling catheters or malignancy. Primary thrombosis of the subclavian and axillary veins constitutes approximately one-quarter of upper extremity deep vein thrombosis. It is thought to occur from compression of the vein as it traverses the thoracic outlet. This compression can be caused by any of the aforementioned anatomic variants associated with neurogenic or arterial TOS. However, like arterial TOS, it is usually due to a cervical rib or the first rib. Compression and potential injury lead to thrombus formation. Often patients report some type of strenuous activity prior to the presentation of symptoms, thus the phrase "effort thrombosis." Symptoms arise from an outflow obstruction and venous hypertension. The treatment of this disease is two-fold. The relief of venous thrombosis is usually performed by thrombolytic therapy. Subsequently, patients are placed on oral anticoagulation for a certain time period to allow endothelial healing, after which thoracic outlet decompression is performed. Unfortunately, some patients can show recurrence during this time. Thus, the ideal waiting period is unclear, but most surgeons usually wait several weeks. Thoracic decompression is usually accomplished by transaxillary or supraclavicular first rib resection. Anticoagulation is then usually continued for approximately 1 month after the procedure. In patients in whom thrombolysis is unsuccessful, operative thrombectomy or bypass can be considered.

Diagnosis

Physical examination

Several maneuvers on physical examination are useful for the diagnosis of TOS. Abduction of the arm from 90° to 180° will usually reproduce the symptoms. Adson's sign involves the loss of the radial pulse on abduction of the arm. This finding is not necessarily reliable, however, as it may occur in a significant number of unaffected individuals[3]. Tenderness over the scalene muscles, brachial plexus, or rotator cuff can be elicited. Rotation or extension of the head can sometimes cause pain in the thoracic outlet region. Patients will also often have a weakened grip. During the later stages, patients can develop muscular atrophy. Specifically, in patients with arterial TOS, evidence of digital ischemia should lead to further testing. In addition, the appreciation of a pulsatile mass along the course of the subclavian artery suggests this disease process. A bruit can also sometimes be heard in this region. Patients with venous TOS present with varying degrees of pain and swelling of the involved extremity. Collaterals of the upper arm, neck, and chest can also appear.

Noninvasive testing

Electromyography
A multitude of neurologic tests are available to evaluate the extremities. Electromyography (EMG) measures motor function. The F-wave response, nerve conduction velocities (NCVs), and somatosensory evoked potentials (SSEPs) measure the response to neural stimuli. For example, SSEPs measure the amplitude of the nerve action potential at particular sites after stimulation of the ulnar or median nerve. Improved SSEPs have been shown to be associated with the treatment of TOS[4]. Nevertheless, these studies are mostly insensitive for the diagnosis of TOS. The sensitivity of these studies does increase, however, with the presence of objective physical findings, specifically extremity atrophy[5].

Pressures and pulse volume recordings
Segmental pressures and pulse volume recordings (PVRs) are used to assess arterial insufficiency. These tests are performed in a similar fashion to lower extremity PVRs (see Chapter 9). Smaller cuffs and lower pressures are used on the digits. Concomitant systolic pressures of the upper extremities are measured in the upper arms, forearms, and wrists. PVRs are taken in multiple arm positions, which can include[6]:
* erect, with the hands in the lap;
* erect, with the arm at a 90° angle in the same plane as the torso;
* erect, with the arm at a 120–180° angle in the same plane as the torso;
* erect, with the arm at a 90° angle in the same plane as the torso and with the shoulders in an extended military-type brace;
* erect, with the arm at a 90° angle in the same plane as the torso and with the shoulders in an extended military-type brace with the head turned sharply towards the monitored arm;
* erect, with the arm at a 90° angle in the same plane as the torso and with the shoulders in an extended military-type brace with the head turned sharply away from the monitored arm.

The test is diagnostic if waveforms flatten in any of the above positions (Figure 11.3). However, it is important to note that a significant proportion of "normal" individuals will demonstrate these findings.

In our vascular laboratory, the same arm positions are used. PVRs are recorded in each of these positions. The elevated arm stress test (EAST) is also employed[7]. The patient elevates both arms at 90° with his or her back against the

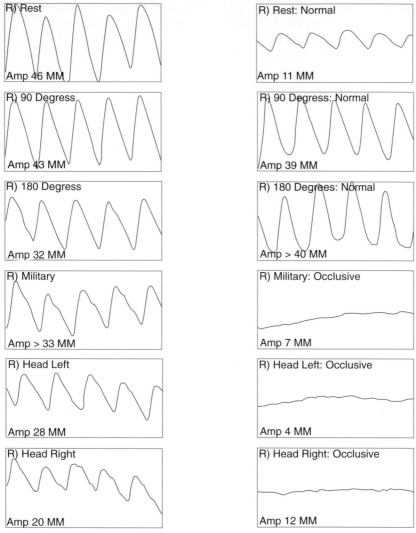

Figure 11.3 Pulse volume recordings of a normal patient (left) and of a patient with thoracic outlet syndrome (TOS) (right). Note the flattening of the waveforms on diagnostic maneuvers.

wall while standing. The patient then open and closes his or her hands for 3 min. If the usual symptoms develop or fatigue results in the arm, TOS may be present.

Ultrasound

Duplex studies are useful for the initial evaluation of suspected venous TOS. It is sometimes difficult to visualize thrombosis of the subclavian and axillary veins. Supraclavicular and infraclavicular approaches are used to assess the subclavian and axillary veins. Color duplex is often used to determine flow pat-

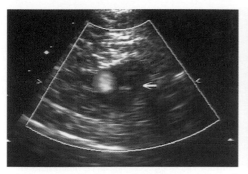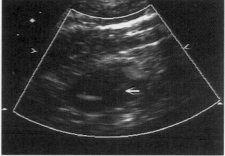

Figure 11.4 Duplex imaging with transverse and sagittal views of nonocclusive deep vein thrombosis of the subclavian vein. Note the filling defects and limited flow (blue) within the vein.

terns as the identification of thrombus by compressive ultrasound is not always easily achieved in this location. Thrombus may also appear as filling defects or as varying degrees of echogenicity (Figure 11.4). Collateral veins are apparent when the subclavian vein is occluded. Finally, evaluation of flow can sometimes identify lesions such as a stenosis. Nevertheless, contrast venography remains the gold standard. Venous thrombosis is easily identified in this manner. Furthermore, compression of the vein as it enters the thoracic outlet can be seen. Even so, appropriate presenting symptoms with a positive duplex study should lead to a high suspicion of venous TOS.

Radiography
Cervical spine films simply entail plain X-rays of the cervical spine region. The presence of a cervical rib can easily be seen. This, however, is not diagnostic of TOS. With symptoms and signs of TOS, a cervical rib may be the cause. However, these ribs can occur in normal patients.

Magnetic resonance imaging
Magnetic resonance imaging (MRI) is useful for the evaluation of the space limitations of the thoracic outlet. Specifically, visualization of the interscalene, costoclavicular, and pectoralis minor spaces can be made during neutral and postural positions. Fibrous bands, narrow spaces, enlarged muscles, compressed vessels, or other anatomic abnormalities can be assessed. Narrowing of the costoclavicular space and arterial compression secondary to fibrous bands in symptomatic patients, in comparison with healthy volunteers, have been noted on MRI[8]. Furthermore, injection of gadolinium can allow the direct assessment of the arteries and veins (Figures 11.5 & 11.6). Thus, MRI provides an adjunctive study to help rule in a thoracic outlet etiology for patients with typical TOS symptoms.

Computerized tomographic angiogram
Computerized tomographic (CT) angiography also provides detailed informa-

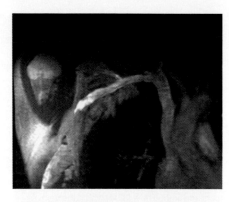

Figure 11.5 Magnetic resonance venogram demonstrating an occluded subclavian vein.

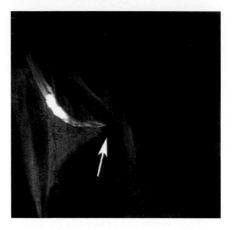

Figure 11.6 Magnetic resonance venogram demonstrating flow limitation of the subclavian vein with complete arm abduction.

tion on the three spaces of the thoracic outlet. As with MRI, it is important to obtain information in both neutral and postural positions. For instance, measurements can be made of the costoclavicular distance with the arm abducted and adducted. When compared with healthy volunteers, symptomatic patients are noted to have a decreased space with postural maneuvers[9]. Furthermore, CT angiography delineates the course of the vessels and any concomitant compression. As with MRI, CT angiography does not provide a diagnosis of TOS, but rather an anatomic correlation in patients with symptoms consistent with the syndrome. It is important to note that anatomic findings suggestive of TOS can be found on axial imaging in normal volunteers[10].

Invasive procedures

A scalene muscle block can be performed by anesthetizing the anterior scalene muscle. This was first described in 1939[11]. If the symptoms and signs resolve, TOS is suspected. The procedure is performed by aiming the needle cephalad over the clavicle into the anterior scalene. Care should be taken not to inject the vascular structures or to cause a pneumothorax. Some have proposed the use of

EMG monitoring to ensure injection in the anterior scalene[12]. This may improve the sensitivity and specificity of the test by reducing "missed blocks." For example, inducing a nerve block could create a false positive result. In contrast, missing the muscle could result in a false negative result.

Venograms are the gold standard for the diagnosis of venous TOS. An appropriate technique is important to obtain an adequate study. The arm must be abducted by at least 30° to allow appropriate visualization. Furthermore, the cephalic vein should not be injected because it directly joins the subclavian vein and bypasses the axillary vein. Arm maneuvers should be performed to recreate any potential venous compression. In general, venography is clearly the best study for visualizing thrombus or venous compression.

In order to diagnose arterial TOS, arteriograms should be employed. Multiple views can be obtained to identify any stenotic regions. As with contrast venography, appropriate arm maneuvers should be undertaken to elicit any lesions that are not obvious at rest. Post-stenotic dilation and aneurysmal changes are also noted. It is also important to visualize the arterial runoff, especially under circumstances in which ischemia may be present. An appropriate therapeutic plan can then be generated from this information.

Finally, intravascular ultrasound (IVUS) has also been employed. In one study, IVUS, which was performed concurrently with venography, was able to identify venous thrombosis in all patients detected by venography[13]. Furthermore, IVUS was employed intra-operatively and aided operative management by demonstrating the resolution of venous compression after simple release of the pectoralis minor.

Conclusion

In general, TOS is often a difficult diagnosis to make. Although neurogenic TOS is more prevalent, arterial and venous TOS are more straightforward and easier to diagnose. A multitude of studies can be employed to aid the diagnosis. However, no individual test can definitively diagnose TOS. Only with careful clinical correlation and corroborating studies can TOS be diagnosed. Ultimately, only the resolution of symptoms after treatment can prove that a patient truly had TOS.

Reference list

1 Sanders R, Cooper M, Hammond S, Weinstein S. Neurogenic thoracic outlet syndrome. In: Rutherford RB (ed.), Vascular Surgery, pp. 1184–1199. Philadelphia: W. B. Saunders, 2000.

2 Schoder M, Cejna M, Holzenbein T, et al. Elective and emergent endovascular treatment of subclavian artery aneurysms and injuries. J Endovasc Ther 2003; 10:58–65.

3 Gergoudis R, Barnes RW. Thoracic outlet arterial compression: prevalence in normal persons. Angiology 1980; 31:538–541.

4 Machleder HI, Moll F, Nuwer M, Jordan S. Somatosensory evoked potentials in the assessment of thoracic outlet compression syndrome. J Vasc Surg 1987; 6:177–184.

5 Cakmur R, Idiman F, Akalin E, Genc A, Yener GG, Ozturk V. Dermatomal and mixed nerve somatosensory evoked potentials in the diagnosis of neurogenic thoracic outlet syndrome. Electroencephalogr Clin Neurophysiol 1998; 108:423–434.

6 Raines JK. The pulse volume recorder in peripheral arterial disease. In: Bernstein EF (ed.), Vascular Diagnosis, p. 539. St. Louis: Mosby, 1993.

7 Raines J. Criteria, Procedures and Instrumentation for the Clinical Vascular Laboratory, pp. 22–23. Greenwich, CT: Life Sciences Inc., 1978.

8 Demondion X, Bacqueville E, Paul C, Duquesnoy B, Hachulla E, Cotten A. Thoracic outlet: assessment with MR imaging in asymptomatic and symptomatic populations. Radiology 2003; 227:461–468.

9 Remy-Jardin M, Remy J, Masson P, *et al.* Helical CT angiography of thoracic outlet syndrome: functional anatomy. Am J Roentgenol 2000; 174:1667–1674.

10 Demondion X, Boutry N, Drizenko A, Paul C, Francke JP, Cotten A. Thoracic outlet: anatomic correlation with MR imaging. Am J Roentgenol 2000; 175:417–422.

11 Gage M. Scalenus anticus syndrome: a diagnostic and confirmatory test. Surgery 1939; 5:599–601.

12 Jordan SE, Machleder HI. Diagnosis of thoracic outlet syndrome using electrophysiologically guided anterior scalene blocks. Ann Vasc Surg 1998; 12:260–264.

13 Chengelis DL, Glover JL, Bendick P, Ellwood R, Kirsch M, Fornatoro D. The use of intravascular ultrasound in the management of thoracic outlet syndrome. Am Surg 1994; 60:592–596.

VI Acquired and Congenital Malformations

12 Complications of Femoral Arterial Vascular Access

Itzhak Kronzon and Paul A. Tunick

Modern technologies for the diagnosis and treatment of cardiovascular disorders frequently require percutaneous penetration into a peripheral artery. The most common point of entry is the femoral artery. Arterial complications are known to occur during diagnostic and therapeutic percutaneous procedures. These complications include bleeding, dissection, infection, thromboembolism, occlusion, arteriovenous fistula (AVF), and arterial pseudoaneurysm (PSA)[1]. The usual technique of femoral artery entry is percutaneous needle puncture with arterial cannulation using the Seldinger technique or some modification of this. At the end of this procedure, after the catheter and sheath have been removed, control of arterial bleeding is obtained by direct pressure. Today's medical economy emphasizes a short hospital stay. Many patients who undergo such procedures are discharged from hospital less than 24 h afterwards. Often there is a subcutaneous groin hematoma which is usually considered to be a minor, spontaneously resolving complication. However, this hematoma may mask more severe complications, e.g. femoral artery iatrogenic PSA and femoral AVF, which, initially, may show no specific symptoms, but may later lead to significant complications. This chapter reviews the clinical aspects, imaging techniques, and therapeutic approach to these vascular complications of arterial access.

Femoral artery pseudoaneurysm

Femoral artery PSA[2–4], also known as false aneurysm, is an extravascular cavity which communicates with the artery through a disruption in the arterial wall. Unlike true aneurysm, which is bound completely by the walls of the artery, a PSA is bound only by local tissue. The PSA comprises two main components: a blood-filled sac and a communication tract or neck which connects the sac to the artery. Characteristically, blood flows from the artery into the PSA during systole, while during diastole blood flows from the PSA back into the artery. The volume of blood that enters the PSA during systole equals the volume of blood that returns to the artery in diastole. In rare cases, when systolic filling is greater than diastolic emptying, this may result in rapid expansion of the PSA with catastrophic complications, such as rupture.

Incidence

Several studies have reported the incidence of PSA detected clinically and/or requiring treatment. A study of nearly 40,000 angiographic procedures by Roberts et al.[5] found an incidence of 0.1% in patients who had undergone diagnostic radiologic angiography and 0.2% in patients who had undergone diagnostic cardiac catheterization. In this group of patients, the mean number of days after catheterization until suspicion of femoral artery PSA was nearly nine. Because small PSAs tend to heal spontaneously at an early stage, and not all of the patients were evaluated systematically for the possibility of PSA, it can be assumed that the true incidence is higher.

Interventional procedures are longer, use larger bore catheters and introducers, and are frequently associated with the administration of anticoagulants or antiplatelet drugs. It is therefore not surprising that the incidence of femoral PSA is much higher after interventional procedures. The incidence in various studies has been reported to be between 3.5% and 5.5%[6,7]. With approximately one million interventional cardiologic procedures performed in the USA every year, an annual occurrence of at least 30,000 femoral PSAs can be assumed. The risk factors for PSA formation have been well described. They include advanced age, faulty technique, inadequate manual compression, concurrent antiplatelet or anticoagulant therapy, large arterial sheath, obesity, hypertension, heavily calcified arteries, and chronic hemodialysis[8–10].

It appears that PSAs are more likely to occur when the puncture site is too low. Two mechanisms may explain the association between the presence of a PSA and low puncture, and the absence of a PSA in common femoral artery puncture. First, the common femoral artery is enclosed (together with the common femoral vein) within the femoral sheath. Peri-arterial hemorrhage is therefore partially limited by tamponade by the femoral sheath, preventing the formation of a PSA. A second mechanism may be associated with the close proximity of the posteriorly located femoral head and superior pubic ramus. This posterior bony support is present during arterial compression after catheter removal. Beyond the common femoral artery bifurcation, there is no bony support and no tamponade by the femoral sheath, and thus there is a higher incidence of bleeding and formation of an iatrogenic PSA. One reason for a low puncture is the difficulty in identifying the location of the inguinal ligament in obese patients. In such patients, the presence of a panniculus results in inferior displacement of the inguinal crease relative to the inguinal ligament. Puncture at the inguinal crease in such a case may result in an arterial puncture below the bifurcation of the common femoral artery[8,9].

Clinical presentation

The clinical diagnosis of a femoral PSA can be made on the basis of the characteristic findings of a pulsatile mass, a palpable thrill, and an audible to-and-fro murmur. Quite often, a femoral PSA is associated with groin swelling or ecchymosis, making the clinical diagnosis very difficult. In fact, many femoral PSAs are first recognized only after a complication has ensued.

Rarely, the first presentation may be rupture (into the retroperitoneal area and, on even rarer occasions, through the skin)[11]. In extreme cases, this may lead to sudden exsanguination and death. Infection of a PSA may produce local signs of inflammation, and sepsis has been reported[12,13]. The PSA may compress adjacent structures. Compression of the femoral vein may cause venous stasis, leg edema, and femoral vein thrombosis. Compression of the femoral nerve may lead to sensory loss or, less frequently, decreased motor function. Rare cases of lower limb compartment syndrome have also been described. Skin erosion caused by focal compression is another unusual complication.

Imaging of femoral pseudoaneurysms

Patients are usually referred for vascular imaging when the physician suspects a PSA on clinical grounds. Many modalities of vascular imaging are very sensitive and specific for the diagnosis of PSA. These include contrast angiography (direct arterial injection of contrast material or digital subtraction after venous injection), computed tomography (CT, with contrast), and magnetic resonance angiography (MRA). Duplex femoral ultrasonography is probably superior to these other techniques. It is noninvasive, less expensive, does not require the use of contrast agents, and is available at the patient's bedside. The proximity of the PSA to the skin permits a wide exposure and an uninterrupted ultrasonographic window. In addition, this proximity allows for the use of high-frequency transducers, resulting in high-resolution images. Doppler studies show the blood flow within the femoral veins, arteries, and the PSA and its communicating tract. The availability and ease of the test are important when recurrent studies are required during the treatment and follow-up of patients with femoral PSAs.

Diagnosis of pseudoaneurysm by ultrasonography

The hallmark of diagnosis is the demonstration of an echo-free space with evidence of swirling blood that communicates with the common femoral artery or one of its branches (Figures 12.1 & 12.2)[14]. This echo-free space is usually, but not always, anterior to the artery, and can be seen in most cases just below the skin, near the site of the arterial puncture. The communication with the femoral artery may have various lengths. In some cases, the communication is almost direct and, in others, the length of the tract may be 2 or even 3 cm between the artery and the PSA. In all cases, however, the diameter of the communication is much smaller than the maximal diameter of the aneurysm. The size of a PSA may vary. It may be as small as a few millimeters and as large as 10 cm in diameter. Not infrequently, partial clotting is noted within the PSA cavity. With the use of high-frequency transducers, swirling spontaneous echo contrast ("smoke") can often be demonstrated.

The flow velocity within the femoral artery, the femoral PSA, and the communicating tract can be demonstrated easily by various Doppler modalities. Color Doppler permits the accurate demonstration of flow within the communication tract and also shows the flow within the aneurysm. Pulsed and contin-

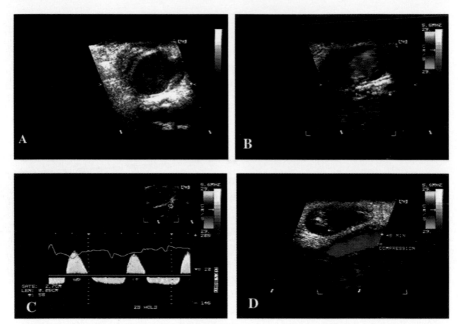

Figure 12.1 Femoral pseudoaneurysm. (A) Note the 2.5 cm × 2.5 cm cavity (PSA) which contains laminated thrombus and spontaneous echo contrast ("smoke") just anterior to the femoral artery (A). The communication tract is just anterior to the artery (arrows). (B) Same as in (A), systolic frame, with color Doppler. Note that there is flow in the artery (blue), in the pseudoaneurysm (red), and also in the tract between them (red). (C) Continuous wave Doppler of the flow in the tract. Flow is to-and-fro, into the pseudoaneurysm in systole (above the baseline) and back into the artery in diastole (below the baseline). (D) After compression and obliteration of the tract, systolic frame, with color Doppler. Note that flow is now limited to the artery and there is no flow in the pseudoaneurysm or tract. (From Kronzon I. Diagnosis and treatment of iatrogenic femoral artery pseudoaneurysm: a review. J Am Soc Echocardiogr 1997; 10:236–245, with permission from Elsevier Publishing.)

uous wave studies can provide further insight into PSA hemodynamics. The direction of flow is from the artery into the PSA in systole and from the PSA back into the artery in diastole[15]. The flow velocity depends on the pressure gradient between the artery and the PSA during the phases of the cardiac cycle. High-pressure gradients are expected in high-resistance communications (narrow, long, serpiginous communication tracts). With wider, shorter tracts, there is a lower pressure gradient and therefore a lower flow velocity. Demonstration of a to-and-fro flow velocity pattern within the communicating tract is an important part of the diagnosis and may also be an important predictor of the response to noninvasive treatment. Three-dimensional ultrasound is a new, evolving technology that allows the demonstration of the entire lesion. With three-dimensional reconstruction, our group has calculated the volume of the PSA and demonstrated the communication with its blood flow in the three dimensions.

During ultrasonography, the entire length of the common femoral artery and

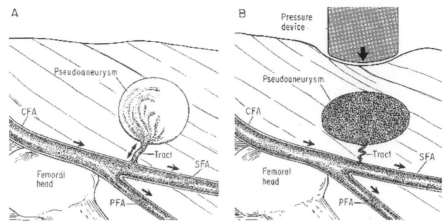

Figure 12.2 Schematic drawing of a pseudoaneurysm compression. (A) Iatrogenic superficial femoral artery pseudoaneurysm. Note that there is a bony support (the femoral head) below the common femoral artery (CFA) but not below the superficial femoral artery (SFA). This may be the reason why the pseudoaneurysm developed (a "low stick"). (B) Compression of the pseudoaneurysm. Note that, with compression, the tract becomes kinked and a clot forms (the pseudoaneurysm becomes a simple hematoma). (From Kronzon I. Diagnosis and treatment of iatrogenic femoral artery pseudoaneurysm: a review. J Am Soc Echocardiogr 1997; 10:236–245, after Fellmeth BD, Roberts AC, Bookstein JJ, et al. Postangiographic femoral artery injuries: nonsurgical repair with ultrasound guided compression. Radiology 1991; 178:671–675, with permission from Elsevier Publishing.)

its main branches should be evaluated. Occasionally, more than one PSA is detected. In addition, other vascular complications may coexist. These include AVF, arterial dissection, intra-arterial clot, and femoral venous obstruction.

Treatment

The traditional, invasive approach to the treatment of femoral PSAs is surgery. However, over the last decade, several new, less invasive therapies have been developed in an attempt to safely and effectively treat femoral PSAs. The two most commonly used nonsurgical techniques, ultrasound-guided compression and ultrasound-guided thrombin injection, have been validated extensively. Other techniques, such as percutaneous vascular stenting and occlusion by coils, have not been used as often but, nonetheless, offer additional innovative nonsurgical approaches to the treatment of femoral PSAs.

Watchful waiting

Several reports in the literature have suggested that a femoral PSA can be safely observed if the patient does not require anticoagulation and if the PSA is small (less than 6 cm^3)[16] and uncomplicated. Some prospective studies have reported spontaneous resolution in 60–93% of patients with observation alone for uncomplicated PSAs. The standard observation procedure requires a weekly physical examination, and ultrasonographic evaluations should be performed until full thrombosis of the PSA is noted[17]. The patient should be advised to avoid strenuous physical activity and to contact his or her physician immediately if pain, swelling, or bleeding occurs[18].

Contraindications to watchful waiting include hemorrhagic, thrombotic, neurologic, ischemic, or infectious complications; large PSA size (> 6 cm^3); an unreliable patient; a long-standing lesion (> 2 months); and required anticoagulation.

Complications which may occur during observation include PSA rupture, limb ischemia, neurologic deficit, arterial or venous thrombosis, embolic phenomena, and pain.

Although no data are available regarding the cost-effectiveness of this approach, frequent office visits and weekly ultrasound evaluations over a prolonged period of time can result in considerable costs. In addition, there is a negative psychologic impact on the patient who has a potentially dangerous vascular abnormality over a prolonged period.

Ultrasound-guided compression

Originally introduced in 1991 by Fellmeth *et al.*, ultrasound-guided compression has gained wide acceptance as a treatment option for PSA because of its proven efficacy, availability, and safety[19–22].

Color flow duplex ultrasonography is used to identify the PSA with the transducer positioned directly above the communicating tract. The minimal force required to arrest flow in the tract is applied. The ultrasound transducer itself is easily used to compress the PSA, and this has an advantage over manual or C-clamp compression in that the flow in the PSA and the tract can be monitored during compression. Analgesia, local anesthesia, and/or sedation may be used if needed. Every 10–15 min, the transducer pressure is temporarily released to evaluate the flow in the PSA. Peripheral pulses are monitored throughout the procedure, and it is important to make sure that blood flow to the leg is not obliterated by the compression (femoral arterial flow can be monitored with the ultrasound transducer). Compression is terminated when thrombosis of the PSA is noted. A post-procedure pressure dressing is usually applied, and a follow-up ultrasound examination is performed in 24–48 h. A mechanical C-arm compression clamp may be used without compromising success rates in order to help relieve the operator of time-consuming, labor-intensive manual compression[19,23].

Contraindications to manual compression include peripheral arterial obstruction, bleeding, arterial or venous thrombosis, limb ischemia, PSA infection, the necessity of occluding the femoral artery in order to occlude the tract, intolerable pain or vasovagal reactions during compression, prosthetic grafts, noncompressible lesions, failure to visualize the communication tract, and lesions above the inguinal ligament.

Complications of compression of a PSA include arterial thrombosis, deep vein thrombosis and pulmonary embolism, limb ischemia, extreme vasovagal reactions, rupture of the PSA, and skin necrosis.

When compared with the high cost of surgical repair and a prolonged hospital stay, ultrasound-guided compression is a cost-effective approach to uncomplicated PSAs. Despite an overall success rate of nearly 75%[19,24], compression has several shortcomings, including a limited success in patients taking anticoagulant or antiplatelet drugs, lengthy compression times (up to 300 min), and considerable recurrence rates (8% overall and 20% for anticoagulated patients)[22].

Ultrasound-guided thrombin injection

There are at least 20 studies that have confirmed the high success rate (95–99%) and low complication rate (1–2%) of ultrasound-guided thrombin injection for the treatment of PSA, even in anticoagulated patients[25,26].

Standard procedure

Under ultrasound guidance, a hypodermic needle is introduced percutaneously into the sac of the PSA. The tip of the needle is positioned away from the communicating tract. Bovine thrombin (500–1000 units; diluted in 1 ml of normal saline) is then injected into the sac. Thrombosis of the PSA usually occurs within seconds but, if it does not, an additional 500–1000 units can be used. The volume of the injection should never exceed the volume of the PSA in order to avoid overflow into the femoral artery. Following successful thrombosis, the femoral artery and vein must be assessed for patency to exclude any distal spillage of thrombin into the native circulation. Distal pulses should be monitored throughout the procedure, and the patient is subsequently kept at bed rest for at least 1 h. A repeat ultrasound is recommended in 24 h. Failure to thrombose the PSA is usually associated with large arterial lacerations, rather than a single puncture site[27].

The complications of thrombin injection are the same as those for compression, but also include failure to visualize the tip of the needle, thrombin spillage into the arterial or venous circulation, and a history of adverse reaction to thrombin or bovine products. Other extremely rare complications include arterial thromboembolism, anaphylaxis[28] or other allergic response to thrombin[29], and disseminated intravascular coagulation (DIC)[30].

Compared with compression, ultrasound-guided thrombin injection provides a significant reduction in the use of vascular laboratory resources, especially with respect to technician time. Moreover, operating room use is reduced, as a lower failure rate means that fewer patients will require surgical repair. Taylor et al.[31] performed a cost calculation at their institution, and found that the average cost per patient was $636 for ultrasound-guided compression and $142 for ultrasound-guided thrombin injection.

In addition to thrombin, other agents, such as collagen plugs, coils, and cyanoacrylate, have been used to thrombose PSAs[4,32,33]. Usually, access to the PSA is accomplished via a percutaneous catheter or direct puncture. However, despite good success rates in several small trials, these agents lack sufficient clinical data to support their use as first-line therapy.

Percutaneous endovascular stenting

Over the past two decades, there have been a number of reports on the use of percutaneous endovascular stenting for the treatment of PSAs.[4] Although the success rate of this procedure is impressive, late stent occlusion has been observed in up to 17% of cases[34]. In addition, unlike compression and thrombin injection, which have been validated by dozens of clinical trials, percutaneous endovascular stenting has not been studied as extensively and should not be considered as primary treatment for PSAs.

A peripheral, balloon-expandable, covered stent is introduced percutaneously into the contralateral femoral arterial circulation and advanced under fluoroscopic guidance to the origin of the PSA. The stent is then expanded by balloon deployment to prevent flow into the communicating tract of the PSA, while allowing normal flow to the distal femoral artery. Within several seconds, thrombosis of the PSA is accomplished. A repeat ultrasound is recommended in 24–48 h, and the patient usually remains at bed rest for at least 4–6 h.

Contraindications to stent placement are the same as those for the other treatment modalities, and also include a small femoral artery and a site of PSA at a bifurcation point.

Complications of stenting include acute or subacute stent thrombosis, late in-stent occlusion, arterial dissection or perforation, distal embolization, stent migration, infection, and groin complications on the contralateral side (another PSA!).

Although endovascular stenting may be less costly than surgical repair, it is not as cost-effective as ultrasound-guided compression or ultrasound-guided thrombin injection. Ultrasound follow-up is indicated immediately and 24 h after the stent is placed, and later as well if complications are suspected.

Surgery

Until the introduction of ultrasound-guided compression in 1991, the traditional approach to PSA was surgery[35,36]. However, with the proven success of both compression and thrombin injection, surgical intervention is mainly reserved for hemorrhagic, thrombotic, neurologic, ischemic, and infectious complications. In addition, patients who have failed less invasive approaches or have been scheduled for a planned surgical procedure involving the groin should be repaired surgically.

The conventional surgical approach involves gaining proximal control of the PSA at the distal external iliac artery, opening the pseudocapsule, and evacuating the hematoma. Nonabsorbable sutures are placed transversely across the puncture site. Some surgeons prefer direct entry into the cavity with digital control of the defect and repair, while others utilize a balloon occlusion catheter to gain proximal control of the artery. If the vessel is severely damaged, formal arteriotomy with endarterectomy and vein patch angioplasty may be required.

Limb ischemia, distal embolization, wound infection, lymphatic damage, femoral neuralgia, and complications commonly associated with general anesthesia and/or delayed mobilization may all be complications of surgical repair.

Surgical repair is not a cost-effective, first-line treatment for uncomplicated PSAs[4]. In general, surgery should be reserved for any PSA associated with hemorrhagic, thrombotic, neurologic, ischemic, or infectious complications.

Femoral arteriovenous fistula (Figures 12.3 & 12.4)

Iatrogenic AVF is another complication of diagnostic and interventional invasive procedures. Abnormal communication between the femoral artery or one of its branches and the femoral vein is created by a needle and frequently further dilated by wires, sheaths, and catheters. The incidence of AVF is significantly lower than that of PSA. It is rare after diagnostic procedures and occurs in approximately 1% of all cardiovascular interventional procedures[37]. Thus, in the USA alone, iatrogenic femoral AVF can be expected in at least 10,000 patients per

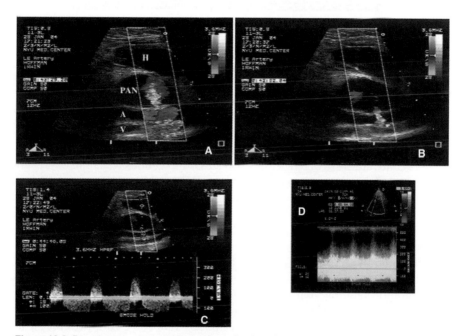

Figure 12.3 Pseudoaneurysm and arteriovenous fistula in the same patient. (A) Systolic frame. This patient has a hematoma (H) just below the skin. Note that there is no flow into the hematoma. Below this is a pseudoaneurysm (PSA). In systole, there is flow from the femoral artery (A) into the pseudoaneurysm. There is also turbulent flow from the artery into the femoral vein below (V). Therefore, this patient has both a pseudoaneurysm and an arteriovenous fistula. (B) Diastolic frame. Note that the blood flow in diastole is from the pseudoaneurysm back into the artery. Flow continues in diastole from the artery to the vein, although it is less than in systole (the pressure gradient from the artery to the vein is less in diastole). (C) Continuous wave Doppler of pseudoaneurysm flow. This tracing also shows the biphasic, to-and-fro flow from the artery to the pseudoaneurysm in systole (above the baseline) and back into the artery in diastole (below the baseline). (D) Continuous wave Doppler of arteriovenous fistula flow. Note that there is continuous, high-velocity flow in one direction (from the artery to the vein). Flow is not to-and-fro, as opposed to that seen in the pseudoaneurysm in (C).

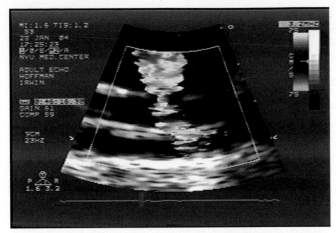

Figure 12.4 Close-up view of the same patient as in Figure 12.3 with both a pseudoaneurysm and an arteriovenous fistula. Note that there is flow from the femoral artery (in the middle) into both the pseudoaneurysm above and the vein below. (Image obtained with a different transducer from that used in Figure 12.3.)

year. The risk factors for AVF have not been well described. As is the case with PSA, a faulty technique, inadequate manual compression, concurrent anti-platelet or anticoagulant treatment, large arterial sheaths, and hypertension may all contribute to delayed healing of arterial and venous wall injury and per-foration, thus leading to persistent communication. Most AVFs arise distal to the bifurcation of the common femoral artery and may involve the superficial femoral artery, the profunda femoris, or its lateral circumflex branch. The fact that most AVFs originate below the bifurcation of the common femoral artery suggests a possible anatomic explanation for the formation of iatrogenic AVFs. The common femoral artery and common femoral veins are located side by side, which makes it difficult to puncture both with one stick. Below the bifurcation, the profunda femoris vein crosses laterally behind the proximal superficial femoral artery and then lies in a posterior location to the profunda. Thus, a lower puncture may perforate both the artery and the vein and create a communica-tion[38]. As mentioned above, one reason for the low puncture is the difficulty in identifying the location of the inguinal ligament in obese patients, which may lead to a lower puncture site[39].

Clinical recognition

The patient may present after cardiac catheterization with a subcutaneous groin hematoma. Palpation may reveal a pulsatile mass. A thrill may also be palpable. Auscultation reveals a continuous murmur which increases in intensity in sys-tole and decreases in diastole (machinery murmur). Even after the hematoma subsides, the skin over the AVF may be warm. Rarely, with a large communica-tion, the lower limb veins appear pulsatile with the development of varicose veins, stasis dermatitis, and ulcers. Congestive heart failure that is reported in patients with other large AVFs (congenital or traumatic) has rarely, if ever, been reported in AVF due to diagnostic or interventional procedures.

As is the case with PSA, all the modalities of vascular imaging are highly specific and sensitive for the diagnosis. However, duplex femoral ultrasonography is the technique of choice. The hallmark of the diagnosis is the demonstration of the communication between the femoral artery and the vein. The vein appears to be dilated and it is frequently pulsatile. There is high-velocity continuous blood flow from the artery to the vein[40]. Continuous blood turbulence is seen within the communication and in the vein. In addition, there is a distinctive type of artifactual extravascular assignment of color, which is more prominent in systole and absent or less prominent in diastole. This artifact may reflect perivascular tissue vibration caused by the turbulent intravascular blood flow. Its presence is helpful in the recognition and the accurate interpretation of the vascular abnormality[41]. Pulsed and continuous wave studies can provide an additional diagnostic insight into AVF hemodynamics. A high-velocity flow jet between the artery and the vein can be demonstrated. For example, with an arterial blood pressure of 120/80 mmHg, and with a venous pressure at the site of the AVF of less than 20 mmHg, the pressure gradient between the artery and the vein will be at least 100 mmHg during systole and 60 mmHg during diastole. Using the modified Bernoulli equation ($\Delta P = 4v^2$), a systolic velocity of approximately 5 m s^{-1} and a diastolic velocity of 4 m s^{-1} would be expected. As with all other iatrogenic damage to the vascular access site, it is important to evaluate the entire length of the artery, including its branches. Not infrequently, more than one communication between the artery and the vein can be depicted. In addition, other vascular complications may coexist, such as PSA, arterial dissection, interatrial clot, and femoral venous obstruction.

Treatment
In an uncomplicated AVF, the prognosis is usually good. Several reports have suggested that serious complications are extremely rare, and therefore this lesion can be safely observed[42,43]. Spontaneous closure is the rule for the majority of observed lesions, but other fistulae have been followed for 4–20 months and have remained asymptomatic. Congestive heart failure due to large AVF has been described, but is extremely rare. Contraindications for observation include associated large PSA, hemorrhage, expanding mass, compromised cardiac output, arterial or venous occlusion, and leg edema.

Ultrasound-guided compression
Ultrasound-guided compression, a procedure similar to that described for PSAs, has also been tried in patients with AVF. There have been several reported successes; however, all the series reported are quite small and the success rate for the obliteration of AVFs is significantly lower than that for the obliteration of PSAs. It appears, however, that approximately 30–50% of all AVFs can be obliterated by compression[44]. The complications and contraindications are very

similar to those described above for PSA. Thrombin injection is contraindicated and should not be used in an attempt to obliterate an AVF for obvious reasons.

Percutaneous endovascular stenting

Several small series have described the utility of covered intra-arterial stenting for the obliteration of AVFs. This procedure is effective; however, late stent occlusion has been reported in up to 20% of patients[34]. The standard procedure, contraindications, and complications are similar to those described previously in the endovascular stent treatment of PSA. Successful occlusion of a symptomatic internal iliac AVF by a venous covered stent has also been reported[45], and may be an alternative to arterial stenting of AVFs.

Surgery

Surgery is relatively safe and is still the most effective approach for the obliteration of AVFs. The complications of surgery have been described above.

Hemorrhage

Hemorrhage is the most common complication of invasive diagnostic and interventional procedures. Major hemorrhage is usually secondary to a large vascular perforation and is associated with large bore catheters and anticoagulation[45]. Faulty technique may result in a low puncture with perforation of the branches of the common femoral artery (i.e. the superficial femoral or the profunda femoris artery) rather than the common femoral artery itself. The branches of the common femoral artery are outside the femoral sheath and therefore the peri-arterial hemorrhage is not limited by tamponade induced by the femoral sheath. A second mechanism is associated with the fact that these branches are away from the femoral head and the pubic ramus, and therefore compression of the artery may not be effective. A short compression period after removal of the catheter or the sheath and mobilization of the patient too early may also be associated with an increased risk of bleeding. Puncture of the external iliac artery (i.e. above the inguinal ligament) may result in bleeding into the retroperitoneal space.

Signs of bleeding include direct visualization of blood spurts through the skin puncture, expanding hematoma, hypovolemia, and shock. The hematoma may be deep, may not lead to ecchymosis, and may present as an enlarging limb. Such hematomas may also compress blood vessels and nerves, and lead to compartment syndrome.

The diagnosis is clinical; however, duplex ultrasonography is sometimes used to evaluate the possibility of vascular injury, such as PSA, AVF, venous occlusion, and arterial dissection or occlusion. The ultrasound examination will frequently show a hematoma as a large collection of blood in different stages of clotting. Unclotted blood may appear hypoechoic, and the presence of PSA must be ruled out. Color Doppler should be used. Obviously, in the case of a simple hematoma, no blood flow will be seen within the hematoma. However, if there is a communication between the artery and the hypoechoic space, blood flow will be demonstrated inside the hypoechoic space (this finding is therefore diagnostic of a PSA).

Treatment includes observation for minor bleeding, and volume replacement and blood transfusion, as well as surgical repair, for severe, continuous bleeding.

Vascular occlusion

Vascular occlusion may be the result of clot formation at the site of the arterial penetration, prolonged occlusion of the artery by compression, or localized dissection induced by an attempt to pass the needle, sheath, wires, or catheters between the layers of the artery. Arterial occlusions are more common in patients with peripheral atherosclerotic disease or small arterial caliber. The signs and findings of acute or chronic limb ischemia, as well as ultrasound and other diagnostic findings, are described in Chapters 9 and 10.

Reference list

1 McCann RI, Schwartz LB, Pieper KS. Vascular complication of cardiac catheterization. J Vasc Surg 1991; 14:375–381.

2 Kronzon I. Diagnosis and treatment of iatrogenic femoral artery pseudoaneurysm: a review. J Am Soc Echocardiogr 1997; 10:236–245.

3 Piedad BT, Kronzon I. Iatrogenic femoral artery pseudoaneurysm. Curr Treat Options Cardiovasc Med 2003; 5:103–108.

4 O'Sullivan GJ, Ray SA, Lewis JS, et al. A review of alternative approaches in the management of iatrogenic femoral pseudoaneurysms. Ann R Coll Surg Engl 1999; 81(4):226–234.

5 Roberts SR, Main D, Pinkerton J. Surgical therapy of femoral artery pseudoaneurysm. Am J Surg 1985; 154:676–680.

6 Kreskowik TF, Khoury MS, Miller BV, Winniford MD, Shamma AR, Sharp JW. A prospective study of the incidence and natural history of femoral vascular complications after PTCA. J Vasc Surg 1991; 13:328–336.

7 Kent CK, McArdle C, Kennedy B, et al. A prospective study of the clinical outcome of femoral pseudoaneurysms and arteriovenous fistulas induced by arterial puncture. J Vasc Surg 1993; 17:125–133.

8 Rappaport S, Sniderman KW, Morse SS, Proto MH, Ross GR. Pseudoaneurysms: a complication of faulty technique in femoral artery puncture. Radiology 1985; 154:529–530.

9 Altin RS, Flicker S, Naidech HJ. Pseudoaneurysm and arteriovenous fistula after femoral artery catheterization: association with low femoral puncture. Am J Roentgenol 1989; 152:629–631.

10 Rocha-Singh KJ, Schwend RB, Otis SM, Schatz RA, Ieirstein PS. Frequency and nonsurgical therapy of femoral artery pseudoaneurysms complicating interventional cardiology procedures. Am J Cardiol 1994; 73:1012–1014.

11 Yan JST. Iatrogenic arterial injuries: damage to femoral artery. In: Greenhalgh RM, Hallier LH (eds), Emergency Vascular Surgery, pp. 232–237. London: W. B. Saunders, 1992.

12 Brummit CF, Kravvitz GR, Franrud GA, et al. Femoral endarteritis due to Staphylococcus aureus complication of percutaneous, transluminal coronary angioplasty. Am J Med 1989; 86:822–824.

13 Krupski WS, Pogany A, Effeney D. Septic endarteritis after percutaneous transluminal angiography. Surgery 1985; 98:358–361.

14 Schwartz RA, Kerns DB, Mitchell DG. Color Doppler ultrasound imaging in iatrogenic arterial injuries. Am J Surg 1991; 163:4–8.

15 Abu-Yousef MM, Wiese JA, Shamma A. The "to and fro" sign: duplex Doppler evidence of femoral artery pseudoaneurysms. Am J Roentgenol 1988; 150:632–634.

16 Paulson EK, Hertzberg BS, Paine SS, et al. Femoral artery pseudoaneurysms: value of color Doppler sonography in predicting which ones will thrombose without treatment. Am J Radiol 1992; 159:1077–1082.

17 Johns JP, Pupa LE Jr, Bailey SR. Spontaneous thrombosis of iatrogenic femoral artery pseudoaneurysms: documentation with color Doppler and two-dimensional ultrasonography. J Vasc Surg 1991; 14:24–29.

18 Schaub F, Theiss W, Busch R, et al. Management of 219 consecutive cases of postcatheterization pseudoaneurysms. J Am Coll Cardiol 1997; 30:670–675.

19 Fellmeth BD, Roberts AC, Bookstein JJ, et al. Postangiographic femoral artery injuries: nonsurgical repair with ultrasound guided compression. Radiology 1991; 178:671–675.

20 Fellmeth BD, Baron SB, Brown PR, et al. Repair of post-catheterization femoral pseudoaneurysms by color flow ultrasound guided compression. Am Heart J 1992; 123:547–551.

21 Hajarizadeh H, La Rosa CR, Cardullo P, et al. Ultrasound-guided compression of iatrogenic femoral pseudoaneurysm: failure, recurrence, and long-term results. J Vasc Surg 1995; 22(4):425–430.

22 Cox GS, Young JR, Gray BR, et al. Ultrasound-guided compression repair of postcatheterization pseudoaneurysms: results of treatment in one hundred cases. J Vasc Surg 1994; 19:683–686.

23 Fellmeth BD, Buckner NK, Ferrira JA, et al. Postcatheterization femoral artery injuries: repair with colour flow US guidance and C-clamp assistance. Radiology 1992; 1182:570–572.

24 Paulson EK, Sheafor DH, Kliewer MA, et al. Treatment of iatrogenic femoral arterial pseudoaneurysms: comparison of US-guided thrombin injection with compression repair. Radiology 2000; 215:403–408.

25 Friedman SG, Pellerito JS, Scher L, et al. Ultrasound-guided thrombin injection is the treatment of choice for femoral pseudoaneurysms. Arch Surg 2002; 137:462–464.

26 Kang SS, Labropoulos N, Mansour MA, et al. Percutaneous ultrasound-guided thrombin injection: a new method for treating postcatheterization femoral pseudoaneurysms. J Vasc Surg 1998; 27:1032–1038.

27 Sheima RG, Mastromatteo M. Iatrogenic femoral pseudoaneurysms that are unresponsive to percutaneous thrombin injection: potential causes. Am J Roentgenol 2003; 181(5): 1301–1304.

28 Pope M, Johnston KW. Anaphylaxis after thrombin injection of a femoral pseudoaneurysm: recommendations for prevention. J Vasc Surg 2000; 32:190–191.

29 Sheldon PJ, Oglevie SB, Kaplan LA. Prolonged generalized urticarial reaction after percutaneous thrombin injection for treatment of femoral artery pseudoaneurysms. J Vasc Intervent Radiol 2000; 11:759–761.

30 Vignolo-Scalone WH, Vignolo-Puglia WH, Kitchens CS. Microvascular alterations in thrombin-induced experimental disseminated intravascular coagulation in the dog. Angiology 1984; 35:261–268.

31 Taylor BS, Rhee RY, Muluk S, et al. Thrombin injection versus compression of femoral artery pseudoaneurysms. J Vasc Surg 1999; 30:1052–1059.

32 Saito S, Arai H, Him K, et al. Percutaneous transfemoral spring coil embolization of a pseudoaneurysm of the femoral artery. Cathet Cardiovasc Diagn 1992; 26:229–231.

33 Hamraoui K, Sjef MP, Pascal FH, *et al.* Efficacy and safety of percutaneous treatment of iatrogenic femoral artery pseudoaneurysm by biodegradable collagen injection. J Am Coll Cardiol 2002; 39:1297–1304.

34 Thalhammer C, Kirchher AS, Uhlich F, *et al.* Postcatheterization pseudoaneurysms and arteriovenous fistulas: repair with percutaneous implantation of endovascular covered stents. Radiology 2000; 214:127–131.

35 McCann RI, Schwartz LB, Pieper KS. Vascular complication of cardiac catheterization. J Vasc Surg 1991; 14:375–381.

36 Roberts SR, Main D, Pinkerton J. Surgical therapy of femoral artery pseudoaneurysm. Am J Surg 1985; 154:676–680.

37 Kelm M, Perings SM, Jax T, *et al.* Incidence and clinical outcome of iatrogenic femoral arteriovenous fistulas: implications for risk stratification and treatment. J Am Coll Cardiol 2002; 40(2):291–297.

38 Sidawy AN, Neville RF, Adib H, Curry KM. Femoral arteriovenous fistula following cardiac catheterization: an anatomic explanation. Cardiovasc Surg 1993; 1(2):134–137.

39 Marsan RE, McDonald V, Ramamurth S. Iatrogenic femoral arteriovenous fistula. Cardiovasc Intervent Radiol 1990; 13(5):314–316.

40 Roubidoux MA, Hertyzberg BS, Carroll BA, Hedgepeth CA. Color flow and image-directed Doppler ultrasound evaluation of iatrogenic arteriovenous fistulas in the groin. J Clin Ultrasound 1990; 18(6):463–469.

41 Middleton WD, Erickson S, Melson GL. Perivascular color artifact: pathologic significance and appearance on color Doppler US images. Radiology 1989; 171(3):647–652.

42 Rivers SP, Lee ES, Lyon RT, Monrad S, Hoffman T, Veith FJ. Successful conservative management of iatrogenic femoral arterial trauma. Ann Vasc Surg 1992; 6(1):45–49.

43 Toursarkissian B, Allen BT, Petrinec D, *et al.* Spontaneous closure of selected iatrogenic pseudoaneurysms and arteriovenous fistulae. J Vasc Surg 1997; 25(5):803–808.

44 Schaub F, Theiss W, Heinz M, Zagel M, Schomig A. New aspects in ultrasound-guided compression repair of postcatheterization femoral artery injuries. Circulation 1994; 90(4): 1861–1865.

45 Cronin P, McPherson SJ, Meaney JF, Mavor A. Venous covered stent: successful occlusion of a symptomatic internal iliac arteriovous fistula. Cardiovascular Intervent Radiol 2002; 25(4):323–325.

13   Doppler of the Hemodialysis Fistula

Mark E. Lockhart and Michelle L. Robbin

Introduction

Hemodialysis in patients with end-stage renal disease requires repeated access to the vessels. Most patients dialyze using a surgically created arteriovenous fistula (fistula) or graft, and access dysfunction is a severe problem. Ultrasound is a useful tool to guide the evaluation and subsequent management of a patient with clinically inadequate dialysis access function. Sonography can often differentiate the etiology of the fistula dysfunction. Etiologies of fistula dysfunction detected by ultrasound include the identification of an anastomotic or draining vein stenosis, large draining vein branches requiring ligation, central venous stenosis, and near or complete fistula thrombosis requiring thrombectomy or a new access site.

Initial placement of a fistula rather than a graft is recommended by the Dialysis Outcome Quality Initiative, when possible, as a result of a fistula's increased longevity and fewer associated infections[1,2]. There has been a recent widespread movement to increase the number of fistulas in use for hemodialysis, with good primary and secondary patency rates. At our institution, we reported an increased frequency of fistula placement based on extensive use of pre-operative mapping (from 34% to 64%), thereby doubling the proportion of patients using a fistula in our population, from 16% to 34%[3]. Despite the optimization of available vessels, many fistulas that are created will not initially mature adequately to support hemodialysis. Patients often undergo hemodialysis for months via a central catheter as they wait for access maturation. Ultrasound can determine the potential etiology of a fistula's failure to develop. Importantly, it can also reduce time wasted on a fistula that will never mature without intervention.

The goals of this chapter are to describe the evaluation of a patient with mature fistula dysfunction and to present in detail the sonographic evaluation of the post-operative fistula for maturation. The anatomy and types of arteriovenous fistula are briefly described.

Types of hemodialysis fistula

Pre-operative sonographic imaging evaluation is a key factor in maximizing a patient's potential for fistula creation[1]. Optimal use of the arm vessels occurs when a fistula can be created in the forearm, saving upper arm vessels for a subsequent fistula. A thigh graft may be used for dialysis if no upper extremity options are available[4]. Hemodialysis with a central catheter is avoided when possible[4], as a permanent access will generally yield higher flow rates[5]. Furthermore, central catheters have significantly higher rates of infection compared with permanent accesses[6]. Catheter-related infections may require repeated catheter exchanges or placement of a new tunneled catheter[7].

When possible, the preferred type of arteriovenous fistula involves the radial artery and the cephalic vein at the wrist or distal forearm of the nondominant arm. The most common type is the Brescia–Cimino fistula, involving an end-to-side anastomosis of the cephalic vein to the radial artery. If the vessels of the nondominant wrist are unsuitable, the dominant wrist vessels are used, when possible. However, a forearm fistula is only possible as the first site of permanent access in 41% of hemodialysis candidates, as a result of vascular problems associated with multiple arterial sticks and venopunctures[8]. Atherosclerotic arterial disease may also limit the successful placement of forearm fistulas.

In many institutions with large diabetic populations, it may be difficult to meet the Dialysis Outcome Quality Initiative recommendation of fistulas representing 50% of new first access placements[2] using only forearm fistulas. After the forearm has been eliminated for fistula placement, attention moves to the upper arm. The preferred site for an upper arm fistula is a cephalic vein–brachial artery anastomosis (brachiocephalic upper arm fistula) near the antecubital fossa. The nondominant upper arm is preferred, similar to the preference of a forearm fistula in the nondominant over the dominant forearm. The caudal aspect of the cephalic vein is anastomosed to the brachial artery to create the arteriovenous fistula. It is necessary to have a small amount of usable cephalic vein immediately below the antecubital fossa to allow the vein to be brought over to the brachial artery. Alternatively, the median cubital vein branching off the cephalic vein is isolated and anastomosed to the brachial artery near the antecubital fossa. The median cubital vein off the cephalic vein must likewise extend to the antecubital fossa so that there is sufficient vein length for anastomosis.

The third type of upper extremity fistula involves a vein transposition, creating a surgical anastomosis of the basilic vein and the brachial artery. As the location of the basilic vein is generally deep and medial, it is inconvenient and difficult to achieve hemodialysis needle placement. Thus, the vein needs to be dissected from its native location and tunneled in the subcutaneous tissues to the antecubital portion of the brachial artery. These tunneled fistulas are generally considered after cephalic vein fistula options have been exhausted, as a result of the extensive surgical mobilization required to move the basilic vein. In some cases, a partially mobilized basilic vein can be anastomosed to the brachial artery without superficialization. However, nonsuperficialized brachial artery–basilic vein fistulas exhibit longer delays until maturation, lower primary success rates, and more complications than their superficialized counterparts. In a high percentage of these patients, a subsequent superficialization procedure assists in the maturation[8]. Therefore, basilic vein fistulas should be performed with primary superficialization of the vein or with the understanding by the patient that a follow-up procedure is likely.

Post-operative fistula assessment

A hemodialysis fistula requires a minimum of several weeks to mature into a high-volume, low-resistance conduit for access. A mature fistula (Figure 13.1) must have a large, palpable vein that allows access with two 15-gauge needles[9]. The fistula should allow a blood flow of at least 300–350 ml min^{-1} for multiple hemodialysis sessions[10,11]. The overall rate of maturation for forearm and upper arm fistulas may be as high as 55–80%[8,10,12–14]. The maturation rate has been reported to be lower in forearm fistulas created based on clinical examination only[13]. The success rate is higher in males and in nondiabetics[10,15,16]. Although

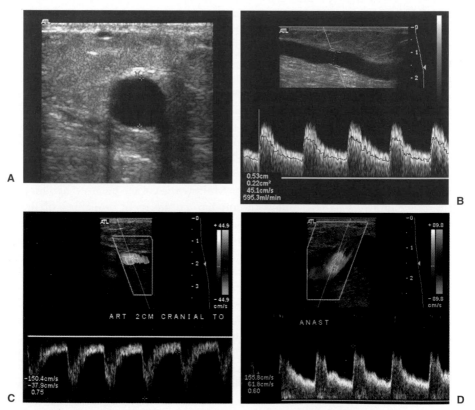

Figure 13.1 Normal mature fistula. (A) Gray scale transverse ultrasound shows that the draining vein measures at least 4 mm in diameter (6.4 mm in this patient) and is less than 5 mm deep. (B) Duplex Doppler shows nonturbulent flow with a low-resistance monophasic arterial waveform and a volumetric flow rate of at least 500 ml min^{-1} in the draining vein. (C) Duplex Doppler 2 cm upstream from the anastomosis shows a peak systolic velocity (PSV) of 150 cm s^{-1}. (D) Duplex Doppler at the anastomosis shows a normal flow with a PSV of 155 cm s^{-1} without a gradient.

diabetes and advanced age may, in combination, increase the risk of fistula failure, there is controversy as to whether age alone should direct a patient to graft placement as a first permanent access rather than attempting a fistula[14,17].

The maturation of an upper extremity fistula is a process that generally requires 2–6 months. If a fistula fails to allow hemodialysis access within 6 months of creation, it is generally considered as having failed to mature. Nonmaturing fistulas are usually difficult to palpate and lack a thrill. Based on the clinical examination of these findings, experienced dialysis nurses are 80% accurate in predicting whether a hemodialysis fistula is mature enough for hemodialysis[18]. In many cases, additional evaluation of a mature fistula with ultrasound is unnecessary if the clinical examination is definitive. However, for a fistula with uncertain maturity based on palpation, ultrasound is a useful noninvasive modality to search for an underlying reason for the apparent nonmaturation. Ultrasound can evaluate fistula characteristics such as the arterial venous anastomosis, vein diameter, and depth from the skin surface. It can also assess for abnormalities, such as draining vein or central stenosis, pseudoaneurysm, and peri-fistula fluid collection.

Indications

Several indications are appropriate for sonographic examination of a hemodialysis fistula. In the first weeks after fistula anastomosis creation, the lack of a palpable draining vein may prompt an evaluation for an underlying etiology for the failure to mature. There are several contributing factors in the failure to mature, including arterial stenosis, venous stenosis, and large branch veins; and ultrasound affords a noninvasive means to visualize these potential abnormalities.

Stenosis of the arteriovenous anastomosis is a major cause of maturation failure, but it may also occur in an established fistula with clinically declining function. A decrease in fistula function is an ominous development, and prompt detection and treatment of any stenosis is important to limit the occurrence of thrombosis. In some patients, the problem may be detected too late with the presentation of a fistula without a palpable thrill. In this case, ultrasound may be useful to document thrombosis for the inexperienced examiner, or in a patient difficult to examine because of obesity or a large hematoma. The detection of a thrombus should prompt appropriate planning for thrombectomy or pursuit of another access site. Ultrasound is indicated in some cases even when a normal thrill and adequate hemodialysis rates are achievable in the fistula. Focal swelling after hemodialysis should prompt an evaluation for outflow stenosis, pseudoaneurysm, or hematoma in these patients.

Ultrasound technique

A relevant clinical history is initially obtained. For sonography, the patient's arm is positioned comfortably on top of a procedure stand with the elbow not quite fully extended. A generous amount of ultrasound gel is used to allow minimal transducer pressure to reduce any vein deformity. A 7 MHz or higher frequency linear ultrasound transducer is used to evaluate the fistula feeding artery and draining vein(s). The feeding artery, arteriovenous anastomosis, and draining vein are examined using gray scale and color Doppler techniques.

Transverse images are obtained to evaluate vessel size and wall thickness. In a forearm fistula, the internal vein diameter is measured in the caudal forearm, mid-forearm, and cranial aspect of the forearm, and at similar levels in the upper arm. In an upper arm fistula, only the upper arm veins require evaluation. The overall minimum diameter of the draining vein is recorded. The depth of the draining vein from the surface of the skin is measured at each level. The vein is followed cranially to check its flow into the deep venous system. The cephalic vein insertion into the subclavian vein is carefully assessed for stenosis or artifact simulating a stenosis. If there is a visible stenosis in the cephalic insertion region, it must be initially viewed with suspicion. It subsequently may have a normal appearance if the arm is placed by the patient's side, instead of the typically abducted position used for insonation.

Color and spectral Doppler evaluation in the longitudinal plane is used to assess for color Doppler aliasing or elevated peak systolic velocities (PSVs) at the arteriovenous anastomosis, or at any visually stenotic area. A tourniquet should not be applied in the routine post-operative examination of an arteriovenous fistula.

Ultrasound evaluation of a hemodialysis fistula must include the subclavian and internal jugular veins. Significant central stenosis or thrombus may hinder maturation of a fistula and limit the usability of a mature access. Color Doppler and spectral evaluation should be performed to characterize respiratory phasicity and cardiac pulsations. The brachial veins should also be examined using compression to evaluate for the presence of thrombus, especially in the patient with unexplained arm swelling.

Established fistula dysfunction: sonographic criteria

Ultrasound is but one method of evaluation for fistula dysfunction. Physical examination, Kt/V [normalized whole-body urea clearance, where K is the dialyzer ability to remove urea (ml min^{-1}), t is the duration of dialysis (min), and V is the volume of urea distribution in the body (ml)], and access recirculation are generally late detectors of a fistula at risk for thrombosis. Accesses may be monitored by ultrasound dilution, pressure measurements, and angiography. However, routine fistula surveillance is not generally performed due to the low incidence of stenosis. A fistula that begins to yield lower dialysis flow rates necessitates sonographic evaluation as a result of the increased risk of subsequent thrombosis or access failure. The most common cause of decreased flow is an arteriovenous anastomotic stenosis. Less commonly, a draining vein stenosis will be the etiology. Likewise, central venous stenosis may lead to access failure if adequate collaterals have not formed.

A normal upper extremity fistula should demonstrate antegrade flow on color Doppler without focal areas of color aliasing or visible stenosis. On spectral Doppler, normal arterial phasic flow with persistent diastolic flow, or a low-

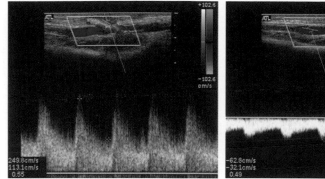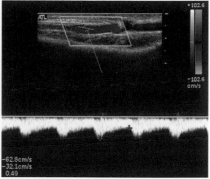

A   B

Figure 13.2 Anastomotic stricture. (A) Duplex Doppler ultrasound of the anastomosis demonstrates color aliasing with a peak systolic velocity measuring 249 cm s^{-1}. (B) The peak systolic velocity in the artery 2 cm upstream from the anastomosis is 63 cm s^{-1}, giving a ratio of > 3 : 1.

resistance waveform, is expected. Although venous tortuosity may be present, a dominant relatively straight venous conduit is usually seen.

Spectral Doppler evaluation of the feeding artery 2 cm cranial to the arteriovenous anastomosis is performed, and the PSV is measured. A similar measurement is obtained at the arteriovenous anastomosis. To assess for a stenosis, a PSV ratio is calculated using the two values as follows: the PSV measured at the arteriovenous anastomosis is divided by the PSV of the feeding artery 2 cm cranial to the anastomosis. If the PSV ratio is three or greater, ≥ 50% stenosis is likely (Figure 13.2)[19]. An attempt should be made to visually confirm the stenosis at gray scale imaging. This is because there may be PSV elevation in the draining vein without the presence of stenosis as a result of the acute angulation of the draining vein off the anastomosis. If the ultrasound is positive for stenosis, the patient is referred for confirmation of the findings on a fistulogram, and angioplasty or surgery. Another specific form of fistula arterial dysfunction is arterial steal, in which the fistula draws too much blood into the draining vein and limits the arterial flow to the hand. This appears on Doppler as reversal of flow in the artery caudal to the anastomosis, and it may be symptomatic (Figure 13.3).

The draining vein is evaluated in a similar manner to the anastomosis, along the entire length of the vein. Color Doppler is useful for the rapid detection of aliasing, which identifies an area suspicious for stenosis. If a draining vein stenosis is suspected visually, PSV is measured 2 cm caudal (upstream) to the stenosis and at the stenosis, similar to the calculation at the anastomosis[20]. A draining vein stenosis is probably present if the PSV ratio is two or greater (Figure 13.4). In some cases, draining vein occlusion may be detected. It typically appears as hypoechoic or heterogeneous thrombus filling the draining vein with the absence of flow on color Doppler (Figure 13.5).

A volume flow rate of 500 ml min^{-1} can be considered as normal, although higher flow rates are often seen, especially in upper arm fistulas. The presence of

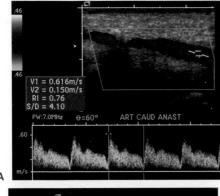

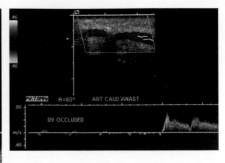

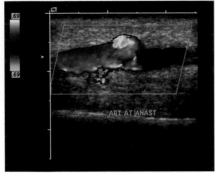

Figure 13.3 Arterial steal. (A) Longitudinal duplex Doppler of the artery caudal to the anastomosis shows the reversal of arterial flow away from the hand. (B) Temporary occlusion of the fistula with gentle pressure results in cessation of flow reversal with little antegrade flow until the compression is released. (C) Color Doppler shows both the proximal and distal aspects of the artery flowing into the fistula.

collateral vessels has been suggested as an etiology for the normal lower flow rates in fistulas compared with grafts[21].

The most common site of fistula stenosis is at or near the anastomosis[22,23]. Treatment of an arterial or venous stenosis may require balloon angioplasty or surgical revision. However, the salvage rate in dysfunctional forearm fistulas can be as high as 95–98%, with 1 year primary and secondary patency rates of approximately 51–62% and 85–86%, respectively[23,24].

Abnormal venous outflow is detected as the absence of the transient reversal of flow in the subclavian or internal jugular vein (Figure 13.6). Monophasic flow in the medial subclavian vein and internal jugular vein that does not return to baseline suggests a central stenosis and should be further evaluated by magnetic resonance venography (MRV) or conventional venography. An exception to this rule is the upper arm fistula with a high amount of flow, in which monophasic flow not returning to baseline may be seen without a central stenosis. A chronic central stenosis may have well-developed collaterals that allow continued function of the hemodialysis fistula. If there is a high degree of clinical suspicion for a central stenosis, an MRV should be obtained even if the ultrasound is negative.

Fistula maturity: sonographic criteria

The failure of fistula to mature is usually due to a vascular stenosis[25]. The spec-

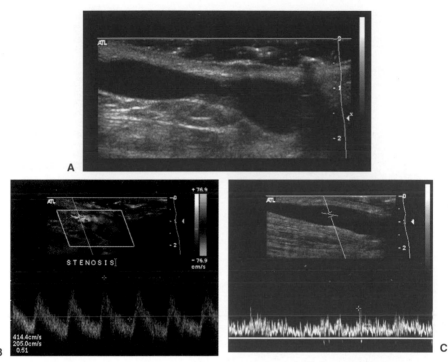

Figure 13.4 Draining vein stenosis. (A) Longitudinal gray scale image shows focal narrowing of the draining vein. (B) Spectral Doppler at the region of narrowing demonstrates high-velocity flow (414 cm s^{-1}). (C) Lower velocity flow (118 cm s^{-1}) is present in the vein 2 cm upstream from the stenosis, yielding a peak systolic velocity (PSV) ratio of 3.5.

tral Doppler criteria for stenosis at a newly created anastomosis are the same as those used for an established fistula (PSV ratio of three or greater at an anastomosis or two or greater in the draining vein). Visual confirmation of the stenosis should be attempted by gray scale ultrasound, because of the acute angulation of the draining vein, as already discussed in the previous section. Velocity criteria in the first few days after fistula creation may possibly be different because of edema and the subsequent venous diameter increase that occurs in response to arterialization of the vein.

The diagnostic criteria that have been specifically associated with fistula maturity are the venous diameter and volumetric flow rate in the venous aspect of the fistula. A draining vein diameter of at least 0.4 cm correlates with fistula maturation. This may be evaluated with a single study in the first 2 months after fistula creation, as the diameter of the vein does not appear to increase after the first 2 months[18]. However, exercise, such as hand squeezing a ball, does increase the fistula diameter, and is often recommended by surgeons after fistula procedures[26]. The venous diameter should be considered in conjunction with volumetric flow determination by spectral Doppler. If the blood flow in the fistula is ≥ 500 ml min^{-1}, there is a high probability of fistula adequacy to allow hemodial-

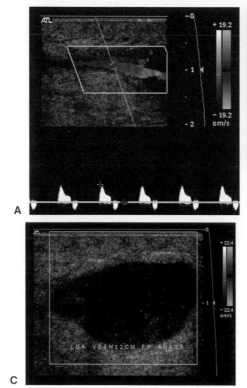

Figure 13.5 Draining vein occlusion. (A) Longitudinal duplex Doppler of the draining vein shows high-resistance antegrade flow with transient reversal of diastolic flow. (B) Color Doppler further downstream in the draining vein demonstrates a small amount of flow in nonocclusive thrombus. (C) Color Doppler further downstream shows expansion of the vein with a hypoechoic clot and absence of flow, consistent with occlusive thrombosis.

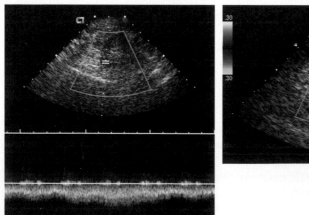
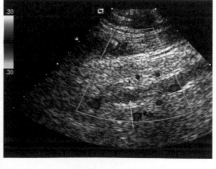

Figure 13.6 Central venous stenosis. (A) Longitudinal spectral Doppler of the fistula shows a small diameter and slow monophasic flow. No anastomotic stricture or large branches were identified. (B) Color Doppler of the subclavian vein shows hypoechoic thrombus (arrow), which can limit fistula maturation.

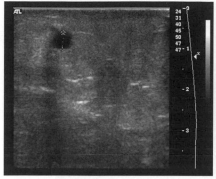
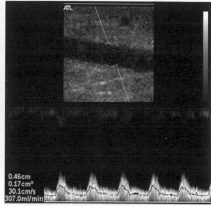

A

B

Figure 13.7 Failure to mature. (A) Gray scale transverse ultrasound shows a small diameter of the draining vein (3.0 mm) that is inadequate for hemodialysis cannulation. (B) The volume flow rate is low, measuring 241 ml min⁻¹. Note that no stricture was identified on duplex Doppler.

ysis, independent of venous diameter. Moreover, the combination of venous diameter and flow volume, using a minimum venous diameter of at least 0.4 cm and a flow volume of at least 500 ml min⁻¹, correlates with a mature fistula in 95% of patients, vs. only 33% success when neither criterion is met (Figure 13.7)[18].

At least one study has evaluated flow rates by ultrasound dilution in the early peri-operative period as a predictor of fistula maturation. It suggested that blood flow is maximal in a fistula as early as 1 week after anastomosis creation and remains constant in the first few months[27,28]. Furthermore, the access flow rates in the early period are predictive of subsequent fistula failure to mature. Patients with low blood flow rates (mean of 450 ml min⁻¹) show greater failure rates than patients with high flow rates (mean of 814 ml min⁻¹)[27].

Occasionally, there may be good flow within a fistula, but the vein may be too deep to access for hemodialysis (Figure 13.8). In the evaluation of a draining vein that is difficult to palpate, the vein depth from the skin surface should be measured by ultrasound. We consider 0.5 cm as the maximum acceptable depth of the vein for access. If the vein is too deep, it may be problematic to palpate the fistula for hemodialysis needle placement[18]. In such cases, the surgeon may be required to superficialize the vein to allow adequate needle access for dialysis if the fistula is otherwise adequate.

In the development of an adequate fistula, large venous branches may draw flow away from the draining vein. Resultant low blood flow in the venous portion of the fistula may contribute to the failure of fistula maturity[22]. We typically consider large branches in the first 10 cm of the vein as the most significant risk to fistula maturation. Surgical ligation can be performed to increase flow in the main vein and improve the likelihood of developing an adequate fistula[29]. Considering all types of salvage procedure, therapeutic assistance of a previously nonmaturing fistula can yield a very high likelihood of a fistula that may subsequently allow dialysis[22].

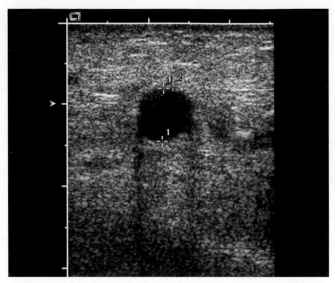

Figure 13.8 Deep draining vein. Transverse gray scale image shows a large draining vein with adequate flow, but the depth of the vein is likely to prevent consistent cannulation. Note that, after superficialization surgery, the fistula was successfully used for hemodialysis.

The criteria for central venous occlusion include venous flow that does not reflect transmitted cardiac and respiratory pulsatility, demonstrated by an absence of a return to baseline at spectral Doppler, identical to findings in an established fistula. If the central veins are evaluated as part of the pre-operative sonographic mapping and no central catheters are placed in the interval, the prevalence of central venous stenosis in the peri-operative period should be minimized. Furthermore, angioplasty of a central venous stenosis can increase flow to allow maturation of the fistula in these situations.

Most of the diagnostic criteria regarding hemodialysis fistulas are based on an evaluation of the anastomosis or draining veins. It should be noted that the presence of peripheral arterial disease (Figure 13.9) correlates with poorer rates of fistula maturation[10]. Early failure has been specifically associated with increased arterial intimal thickness. In one-half of patients with intimal hyperplasia, there was early fistula failure, compared with no early failures in 14 patients without intimal hyperplasia[30].

Conclusions

Color and spectral Doppler are invaluable means of detecting an etiology for arteriovenous fistula dysfunction, of characterizing the reason for failure to mature, and of detecting central venous thrombosis. It is hoped that ongoing work in this area will decrease the need for dialysis by a tunneled catheter and lessen the time a patient must wait for a functional hemodialysis access.

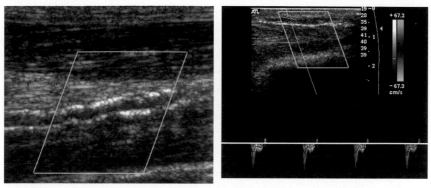

A   B

Figure 13.9 Intimal hyperplasia of the radial artery. (A) Longitudinal color Doppler image of the radial artery shows concentric wall thickening with echogenic calcifications. (B) Duplex Doppler demonstrates high resistance in areas of narrowing within the artery. Arterial insufficiency is one etiology for fistula failure to mature.

Acknowledgments

We would like to thank Trish Thurman for her assistance with manuscript preparation. We would also like to acknowledge the invaluable time and dedication of the sonographers at the University of Alabama at Birmingham and The Kirklin Clinic, our hemodialysis access program, and our ultrasound radiology assistant, Michael Clements, BS, RDMS, RVT.

Reference list

1 Allon M, Robbin ML. Increasing arteriovenous fistulas in hemodialysis patients: problems and solutions. Kidney Int 2002; 62:1109–1124.

2 National Kidney Foundation. K/DOQI Clinical Practice Guidelines for Vascular Access, 2000. Am J Kidney Dis 2001; 37(Suppl. 1):S137–S181.

3 Allon M, Lockhart ME, Lilly RZ, et al. Effect of preoperative sonographic mapping on vascular access outcomes in hemodialysis patients. Kidney Int 2001; 60(5):2013–2020.

4 Miller CD, Robbin ML, Barker J, et al. Comparison of arteriovenous grafts in the thigh and upper extremities in hemodialysis patients. J Am Soc Nephrol 2003; 14(11):2942–2947.

5 Moss AH, Vasilakis C, Holley JL, et al. Use of a silicone dual-lumen catheter with a dacron cuff as a long-term vascular access for hemodialysis patients. Am J Kidney Dis 1990; 16(3):211–215.

6 Fan PY, Schwab SJ. Vascular access: concepts for the 1990s. J Am Soc Nephrol 1992; 3(1):1–11.

7 Tanriover B, Carlton D, Saddekni S, et al. Bacteremia associated with tunneled dialysis catheters: comparison of two treatment strategies. Kidney Int 2000; 57:2151–2155.

8 Fitzgerald JT, Schanzer A, Chin AI, et al. Outcomes of upper arm arteriovenous fistulas for maintenance hemodialysis access. Arch Surg 2004; 139:201–208.

9 Beathard GA. Physical examination of the dialysis vascular access. Semin Dialysis 1998; 11:231–236.

10 Obialo CI, Tagoe AT, Martin PC, et al. Adequacy and survival of autogenous arteriovenous fistula in African American hemodialysis patients. ASAIO J 2003; 49(4):435–439.

11 Miller PE, Tolwani A, Luscy CP, *et al.* Predictors of adequacy of arteriovenous fistulas in hemodialysis patients. Kidney Int 1999; 56(1):275–280.

12 Murphy GJ, Saunders R, Metcalfe M, *et al.* Elbow fistulas using autogenous vein: patency rates and results of revision. Postgrad Med J 2002; 78(922):483–486.

13 Hakaim AG, Nalbandian M, Scott T. Superior maturation and patency of primary brachio-cephalic and transposed basilic vein arteriovenous fistulae in patients with diabetes. J Vasc Surg 1998; 27(1):154–157.

14 Lin SL, Huang CH, Chen HS, *et al.* Effects of age and diabetes on blood flow rate and primary outcome of newly created hemodialysis arteriovenous fistulas. Am J Nephrol 1998; 18(2):96–100.

15 Allon M, Ornt DB, Schwab SJ, *et al.* Factors associated with the prevalence of arteriovenous fistulas in hemodialysis patients in the HEMO study. Kidney Int 2000; 58(5):2178–2185.

16 Golledge J, Smith CJ, Emery J, *et al.* Outcome of primary radiocephalic fistula for haemodialysis. Br J Surg 1999; 86(2):211–216.

17 Windus DW, Jendrisak MD, Delmez JA. Prosthetic fistula survival and complications in hemodialysis patients: effects of diabetes and age. Am J Kidney Dis 1992; 19(5):448–452.

18 Robbin ML, Chamberlain NE, Lockhart ME, *et al.* Hemodialysis arteriovenous fistula maturity: US evaluation. Radiology 2002; 225(1):59 61.

19 Lockhart ME, Robbin ML. Hemodialysis access ultrasound. Ultrasound Q 2001; 17(3):157–167.

20 Robbin ML, Oser RF, Allon M, *et al.* Hemodialysis access graft stenosis: US detection. Radiology 1998; 208:655–661.

21 Bay WH, Henry ML, Lazarus JM, *et al.* Predicting hemodialysis access failure with color flow Doppler ultrasound. Am J Nephrol 1998; 18(4):296–304.

22 Beathard GA. Aggressive treatment of early fistula failure. Kidney Int 2003; 64(4):1487–1494.

23 Rajan DK, Bunston S, Misra S, *et al.* Dysfunctional autogenous hemodialysis fistulas: outcomes after angioplasty—are there clinical predictors of patency. Radiology 2004; 232(2): 508–515.

24 Turmel-Rodrigues L, Pengloan J, Baudin S, *et al.* Treatment of stenosis and thrombosis in haemodialysis fistulas and grafts by interventional radiology. Nephrol, Dialysis, Transplant 2000; 15(12):2029–2036.

25 Turmel-Rodrigues L, Mouton A, Birmelé B, *et al.* Salvage of immature forearm fistulas for haemodialysis by interventional radiology. Nephrol, Dialysis, Transplant 2001; 16: 2365–2371.

26 Oder TF, Teodorescu V, Uribarri J. Effect of exercise on the diameter of arteriovenous fistulae in hemodialysis patients. ASAIO J 2003; 49(5):554–555.

27 Kim YO, Yang CW, Yoon SA, *et al.* Access blood flow as a predictor of early failures of native arteriovenous fistulas in hemodialysis patients. Am J Nephrol 2001; 21(3):221–225.

28 Begin V, Ethier J, Dumont M, *et al.* Prospective evaluation of the intra-access flow of recently created native arteriovenous fistulae. Am J Kidney Dis 2002; 40(6):1277–1282.

29 Miller CD, Robbin ML, Allon M. Gender differences in outcomes of arteriovenous (A-V) fistulas in hemodialysis patients. Kidney Int 2003; 63(1):346–352.

30 Kim YO, Song HC, Yoon SA, *et al.* Preexisting intimal hyperplasia of radial artery is associated with early failure of radiocephalic arteriovenous fistula in hemodialysis patients. Am J Kidney Dis 2003; 41(2):422–428.

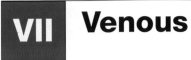

PART VII

VII Venous

14 Upper Extremity Venous Ultrasonography

Marie Gerhard-Herman

Upper extremity venous thrombosis

Upper extremity venous thrombosis includes venous thrombosis of the internal jugular, subclavian, axillary, and upper arm veins. The consequences of upper extremity deep vein thrombosis may include pulmonary embolism in up to one-third of patients[1]. The incidence of upper extremity deep vein thrombosis has increased dramatically coincident with the increasing use of central venous catheters and pacemaker and defibrillator leads[2–4]. Catheter-related thrombosis occurs secondary to vein wall microtrauma, which activates the coagulation cascade. It may occur in the setting of hypercoagulable states, such as malignancy. Repeated trauma to the vein wall with positional thoracic outlet obstruction also leads to subclavian and axillary venous thrombosis.

Primary upper extremity venous thrombosis is unusual, and is commonly divided into two categories[5]: idiopathic or effort thrombosis (Paget–Schoroetter syndrome). Effort thrombosis occurs in the subclavian veins of the dominant arm in an otherwise young, healthy patient after strenuous repetitive exertion involving the upper extremities, such as rowing or weight lifting (see Chapter 11). Effort thrombosis may also be secondary to vein wall microtrauma.

Upper extremity venous anatomy

Ultrasonography is an easily accessible testing modality for the evaluation of upper extremity venous thrombosis. The venous evaluation typically proceeds from the neck to the medial aspect of the clavicle and then laterally to the arm, stopping at the antecubital fossa (Figure 14.1). The internal jugular, subclavian, axillary, basilic, brachial, and cephalic veins are evaluated. At the medial aspect of the clavicle, the subclavian vein joins the internal jugular vein to form the brachiocephalic vein. The subclavian vein becomes the axillary vein as it crosses the first rib. The subclavian, axillary, and brachial veins are paired with arteries of the same name. The basilic and cephalic veins are superficial veins and do not have associated arteries. The basilic vein joins the axillary vein medially at the level of the axilla. The cephalic vein is located on the lateral aspect of the upper arm and joins the venous system more proximally, where the axillary vein becomes the subclavian vein.

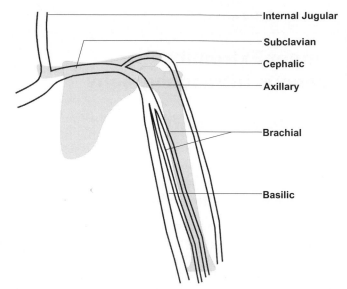

Internal Jugular

Subclavian

Cephalic

Axillary

Brachial

Basilic

Figure 14.1 Veins of the upper extremity. These veins in the neck, upper chest, and upper arm are routinely evaluated during upper extremity ultrasound.

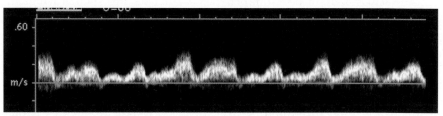

Figure 14.2 Spectral Doppler venous waveform. Velocities vary throughout the respiratory and cardiac cycles in response to changes in intrathoracic and intracardiac (right heart) pressures.

Examination of upper extremity veins

Duplex examination typically begins with transverse gray scale imaging of the internal jugular vein. Spectral Doppler evaluation of the venous waveform is performed at all sites throughout the upper extremity (Figure 14.2). Gentle compression is intermittently applied to evaluate whether the vein can be completely compressed, without compressing the ipsilateral carotid artery (Figure 14.3). The vein is evaluated from the mandible to the clavicle. The sample volume is placed center stream with the cursor parallel to the wall and at a 60° angle with respect to the insonation beam. As velocity measurement is not performed on the venous examination, the angle of insonation is not as important as with arterial ultrasonography, but a 60° angle provides for an acceptable spectral waveform. Spectral and color Doppler are utilized to identify the subclavian vein both above and below the clavicle (Figure 14.4). The subclavian

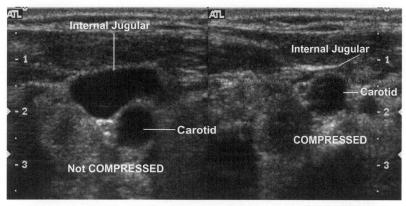

Figure 14.3 Normal compressibility of the internal jugular vein. The vein is seen fully distended in transverse imaging on the left, and compressed in the panel on the right.

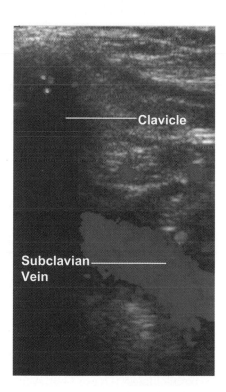

Figure 14.4 Color Doppler examination of the subclavian vein. The subclavian vein has a color Doppler flow signal filling the entire lumen. Acoustic shadowing from the clavicle limits the ultrasound interrogation in this region.

vein within the bony thorax cannot be compressed. Evaluation of this segment relies solely on Doppler evaluation and assessment for venous collapse with rapid inspiration or sniffing. The distal subclavian vein and the axillary veins are then evaluated in the transverse position with gentle compression. Transverse images of the upper extremity veins, with and without gentle compres-

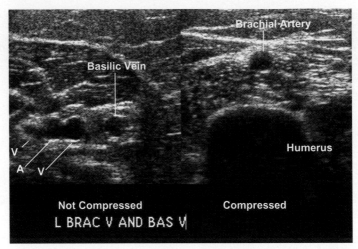

Figure 14.5 Transverse imaging of the brachial and basilic veins in the medial upper arm. On the left, the brachial veins are evident on either side of the brachial artery, while the basilic vein does not have a paired artery. Only the brachial artery is evident in the right panel, which was obtained during gentle compression.

sion, are recorded throughout the axilla and upper arm. The brachial veins are deep and central in the upper arm, and will be present on either side of the brachial artery. The brachial veins are normally easily compressible without compressing the brachial artery (Figure 14.5). The basilic vein is also evident in transverse medial imaging of the upper arm. The cephalic vein is lateral in the upper arm. Pulsed wave Doppler evaluation is performed in the longitudinal plane of all the upper extremity veins. There is normally variation in the waveform in response to respiration and changes in intrathoracic pressures[6].

Diagnosis of venous thrombosis

Venous thrombosis is diagnosed when the vein cannot be completely compressed (Figure 14.6). This is not possible in the proximal subclavian vein. In this location, venous thrombosis is suggested when there is echogenic material within the lumen, incomplete color Doppler filling of the lumen (Figure 14.7), or absence of venous collapse with abrupt sniffing[7]. Thrombosis proximal to the subclavian vein is suggested if the venous waveform lacks variation with respiration. Catheters are visible within the vein as linear structures composed of parallel lines[8] (Figure 14.8). A thin, double-walled linear structure may be evident after catheter removal and is referred to as the "fibrin sheath." Venous thrombosis is present if the vein is not completely compressible around the catheter or fibrin sheath (Figure 14.9). Doppler flow should be detectable around catheters and pacemaker leads in the central vessels. If no flow is detected, central venous thrombosis should be suspected. Thrombus is echolucent when it is acute, and becomes echogenic as it ages. Acute venous thrombosis

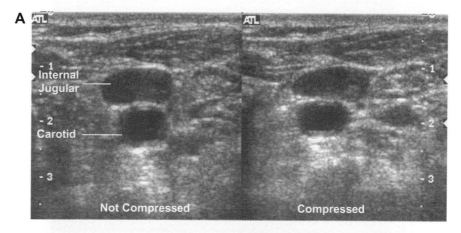

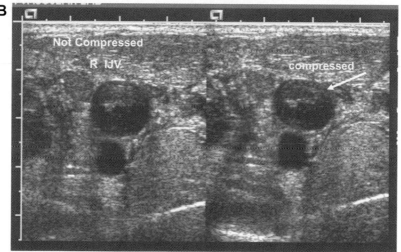

Figure 14.6 Internal jugular venous thrombosis. The examination format records images without gentle compression on the left and with gentle compression on the right. In both cases, the internal jugular vein does not compress. The internal jugular vein thrombus in (A) is more echolucent than that in (B). Therefore, the internal jugular vein thrombosis in (A) is likely to be the most acute. The echolucent noncompressible material in the vein is also thrombus. Echogenic material (arrow) is also evident. Thrombus becomes more echogenic as it ages.

may dilate and distend the vein. The vein size decreases as the vein remodels and the thrombus retracts in the presence of persistent venous thrombosis.

Malignancy

Renal cell carcinoma and other solid tumors exhibit tropism for the intravascular space. These tumors can be seen within the veins of the upper extremity. In contrast with venous thrombus, Doppler evaluation will identify arterial flow

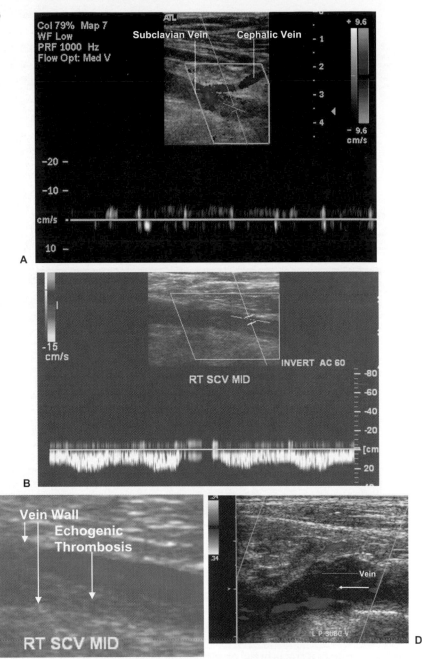

Figure 14.7 Subclavian vein thrombosis. (A) There is no color Doppler signal present through most of the vein. Spectral Doppler evaluation is used to confirm the lack of flow. (B) The spectral Doppler signal is blunted, suggesting that more proximal obstruction to flow is present. This Doppler signal should be compared with the spectral Doppler signals from the contralateral side to determine whether the obstruction to flow affects one or both sides. (C) Color Doppler does not fill the lumen, and echogenic material is evident within the lumen. These findings are consistent with subclavian vein thrombosis. (D) The subclavian vein appears distended, and color Doppler does not fill the lumen. The echogenic material is consistent with thrombus.

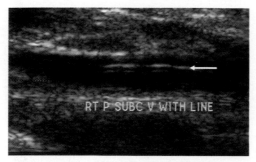

Figure 14.8 Subclavian venous catheter. The catheter is visible as a double-walled structure. There may be additional parallel lines seen as a result of ring down artifact.

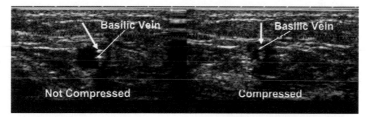

Figure 14.9 Fibrin sheath. The parallel lines (arrow) of the fibrin sheath are present following the removal of a long-term, indwelling venous catheter. The vein is not entirely compressible around the fibrin sheath, consistent with the presence of venous thrombosis in association with the sheath.

Figure 14.10 Renal cell carcinoma metastatic to the internal jugular vein. (A) Echogenic material is seen within the lumen of the internal jugular vein in the longitudinal plane. (B) This material appears to be extending through the wall on transverse images. (C) Power Doppler (arrows) indicates a vascular pattern within the echogenic material, consistent with tumor. *(Continued on p. 182.)*

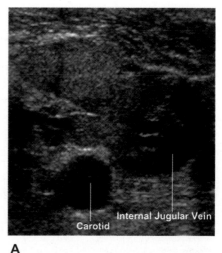

A

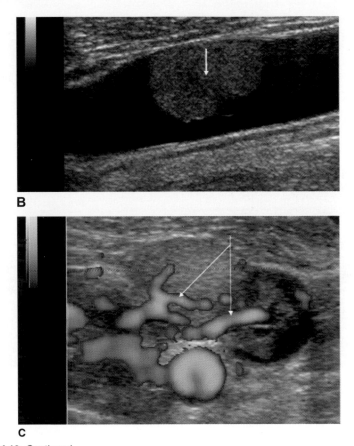

B

C

Figure 14.10 *Continued*

within the intraluminal mass (Figure 14.10). Tumors within the chest may also compress the central veins. A common clinical presentation of this is superior vena cava syndrome. It has also been suggested that upper extremity venous thrombosis is a stronger predictor of occult malignancy than is deep vein thrombosis of the lower extremities[9].

Reference list

1 Prandoni P, Polistena P, Bernardi E, *et al*. Upper-extremity deep vein thrombosis. Risk factors, diagnosis, and complications. Arch Intern Med 1997; 157:57–62.
2 Horattas MC, Wright DJ, Fenton AH, *et al*. Changing concepts of deep venous thrombosis of the upper extremity—report of a series and review of the literature. Surgery 1988; 104:561–567.
3 Joffe HV, Goldhaber SZ. Upper-extremity deep vein thrombosis. Circulation 2002; 106:1874–1880.

4 Kommareddy A, Zaroukian MH, Hassouna HI. Upper extremity deep venous thrombosis. Semin Thromb Hemost 2002; 28:89–99.
5 Becker DM, Philbrick JT, Walker FBT. Axillary and subclavian venous thrombosis. Prognosis and treatment. Arch Intern Med 1991; 151:1934–1943.
6 Rose SC, Kinney TB, Bundens WP, Valji K, Roberts AC. Importance of Doppler analysis of transmitted atrial waveforms prior to placement of central venous access catheters. J Vasc Intervent Radiol 1998; 9:927–934.
7 Grassi CJ, Polak JF. Axillary and subclavian venous thrombosis: follow-up evaluation with color Doppler flow US and venography. Radiology 1990; 175:651–654.
8 Burbidge SJ, Finlay DE, Letourneau JG, Longley DG. Effects of central venous catheter placement on upper extremity duplex US findings. J Vasc Intervent Radiol 1993; 4:399–404.
9 Girolami A, Prandoni P, Zanon E, Bagatella P, Girolami B. Venous thromboses of upper limbs are more frequently associated with occult cancer as compared with those of lower limbs. Blood Coagul Fibrinolysis 1999; 10:455–457.

15 Lower Extremity Venous Ultrasonography

John Gocke

Introduction

Venous disease, including deep vein thrombosis (DVT), pulmonary embolism (PE), varicose veins (Vv), and chronic venous insufficiency (CVI), is the most common vascular disease to afflict mankind, at least in developed countries in which epidemiologic data are available. The reported annual incidences of DVT and PE are in the ranges 44–145 and 21–65 per 100,000 population in the USA[1-5]. Varicosities have been reported to be prevalent in 20–25% of women and 10–15% of men in many countries[6-8], and venous thromboembolism (VTE) in the USA occurs for the first time in Americans at a rate of over 200,000 new cases each year[9,10]. Of these first-time cases, approximately one-quarter of patients will die within 7 days of VTE onset. Because of the large burden of morbidity, mortality, disability, and disfigurement that venous disease places on the general population, I have been very interested in the early and accurate diagnosis of venous disease for a number of years.

I have had the privilege of witnessing first-hand over the past 25 years the astounding migration from venography[11] to continuous wave (CW) Doppler[12-14], phleborheography[15], and impedance plethysmography (IPG)[16-19], and then on to the current gold standard of venous duplex ultrasonography (VDU)[20-24], as the initial diagnostic test of choice for DVT. A strong case can be made that, because of the development of VDU during this same time frame, the ease and rapidity of making a DVT diagnosis has been markedly enhanced. Certainly, the availability of an initial diagnostic test meeting both patient and clinician acceptance has increased, and the risk to the patient of the first-line test has decreased compared with venography. Most importantly, for the entire population of patients at risk for VTE, VDU provides a more readily available and accurate test than that accessible 25 years ago, raising the overall accuracy of the initial assessment of the at-risk patient population. I particularly remember well both my amazement of the VDU technique on first witnessing its demonstration and my prediction that venous disease management was on the threshold of a revolution after seeing, for the first time, an early video demonstration of VDU by Gail Sandager, RN, RVT, at an ultrasound conference in Chicago in 1984. Such initial reports and other small series[25,26] describing the exciting possibilities offered by VDU were later followed by prospective data[20-22] validating VDU as the preferred diagnostic modality for the assessment of DVT. In the last 10 years, the application of VDU has been expanded into the assessment and management of patients with CVI, which is also discussed in this chapter. With this background, the anatomic details pertinent to venous disease are reviewed, followed by a discussion of the indications, technique, instrumentation, interpretation, and nuances of venous duplex imaging.

Venous anatomy

Much has been learned about venous anatomy since the advent of VDU in the 1980s. Prior to this, the gold standard of venous imaging was contrast venography, which focused mainly on the deep venous structures for pathologic condition identification. One advantage of VDU over venography is that it demonstrates not only the venous lumens (Figure 15.1), but their valvular anatomy, surrounding anatomic structures (Figure 15.2), and fascial layers[25]. In addition, when used in real time, imaging yields functional information regarding the competency or insufficiency of venous valves (Figure 15.3).

Superficial veins of the lower extremity

Generally speaking, while deep veins accompany their matching arteries in both the upper and lower extremities, superficial veins are organized largely independent of major arterial flow. The superficial veins of the lower extremities ultimately drain into either the greater saphenous vein (GSV) or the lesser saphenous vein (LSV). The LSV may have a thigh extension named the vein of Giacomini.

Recently, through the use of VDU, the superficial fascia has also been confirmed to exist; as Bailly first described in 1993, the saphenous vein in the thigh

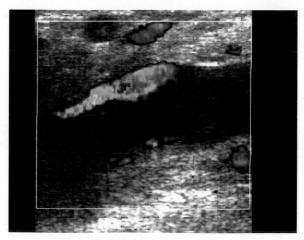

Figure 15.1 Acute deep vein thrombosis with rim of flow.

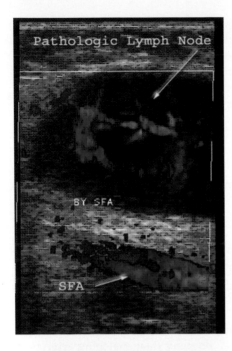

Figure 15.2 Pathologic lymph node.

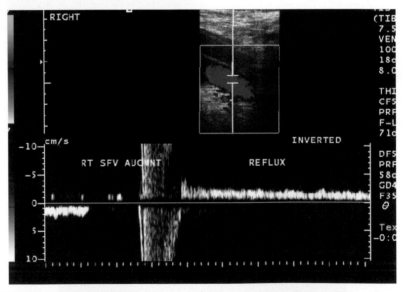

Figure 15.3 Deep vein insufficiency.

sits between the superficial fascia and the deep muscular fascia, and the main trunk may be said to be part of the "Egyptian Eye" in which the saphenous lumen is the iris, the superficial fascia the superior eyelid, and the deep fascia the inferior eyelid[27]. An accessory saphenous vein, which may be a branch of the

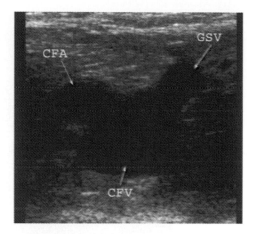

Figure 15.4 Common femoral vein (CFV) at the saphenofemoral junction with the common femoral artery (CFA). GSV = greater saphenous vein.

GSV, may also lie in the upper third of the thigh lateral to the usual location of the GSV. The saphenofemoral junction (SFJ) (Figure 15.4) exists at the inguinal area and represents one of the major connections between the superficial and the deep venous systems. This anatomic site is quite constant, whereas the saphenopopliteal junction, which connects the LSV to the popliteal vein, may be quite variable and may exist anywhere from near the popliteal fossa up to the mid-posterior thigh. The saphenopopliteal junction connecting the LSV to the popliteal vein may not actually exist or be the site of the LSV connection to the deep system in up to 26% of cases; in these cases, the LSV may actually be found to connect to a gastrocnemius vein before entering the popliteal fossa.

Two important proximal venous collaterals of the GSV may be quite large and prominent. The most lateral of the two may be present in 40% of subjects, is called the anterior accessory saphenous vein, and most often joins the GSV very close to the SFJ. The medial collateral often joins the GSV at variable distances and sometimes distal to the GSV valve closest to the SFJ. This vein may actually continue down the posterior thigh to connect with the LSV and become the vein of Giacomini[27].

Deep venous anatomy

The deep veins of the lower extremity below the knee are located deep within the muscle fascias, and are therefore subject to pressure variations that occur with contraction of the calf muscle pump[28]. The deep venous structures of the calf include a pair of posterior tibial veins and the peroneal veins (Figure 15.5), as well as the anterior tibial veins. The gastrocnemius veins and the soleal sinus complexes supply the venous drainage from within the deep calf muscles themselves, such as the gastrocnemius. These deep calf veins all eventually flow into the popliteal vein. The popliteal and the femoral veins are extrafascial and serve as a collecting system conducting the distal lower extremity venous flow from the calf through the thigh and into the pelvis. The external iliac vein begins at the

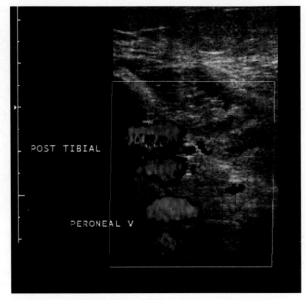

Figure 15.5 Anatomic relationship of posterior tibial and peroneal veins.

inguinal level and drains cephalad into the common iliac vein, which, in turn, drains into the inferior vena cava.

Perforating veins of the lower extremity

Other important connections between the deep venous system and the superficial venous system are the perforating veins. In terms of clinical significance, they are Cockett's veins (Figure 15.6), Boyd's veins near the knee, and Dodd's perforating veins in the thigh (Figure 15.7). In the normal physiologic state, blood flows from the superficial veins through the perforating veins towards the deep venous system. This predisposes that the valve structures within the perforating veins remain competent. In pathologic states in which the perforating veins become incompetent, these perforators appear to become enlarged (Figure 15.8) and demonstrate reflux (Figure 15.9), evidenced by augmented flow passing from the deep system towards the superficial veins. Perforating veins in the normal physiologic state do not usually exceed 1–3 mm in diameter, and may not be readily observable on duplex spontaneously unless there is perforating vein incompetence. Cockett's veins may be involved with worsening venous stasis changes near the medial malleolar regions. Focal intense skin changes overlying perforating vein locations may be intense at times and may actually lead to "perforator blowout" ulceration (Figure 15.10). Thus, careful ultrasound examination of the superficial systems and both the deep and perforating vein systems is essential in a thorough evaluation of venous reflux or venous insufficiency.

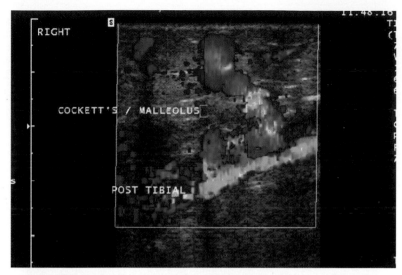

Figure 15.6 Cockett's perforator.

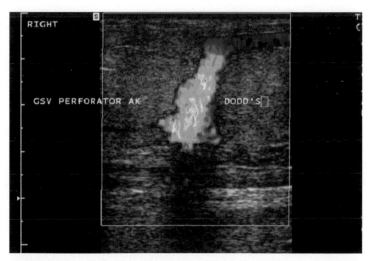

Figure 15.7 Dodd's perforator.

Indications for venous duplex testing

Generally accepted indications for the use of VDU include the evaluation of patients for symptomatic and asymptomatic venous obstruction and venous insufficiency, and the need for venous mapping prior to surgical procedures that will use vein segments as vascular conduits[29]. The assessment of arteriovenous fistulas (Figure 15.11), whether traumatic, therapeutic, or iatrogenic, is also an

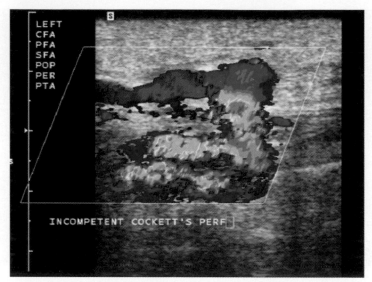

Figure 15.8 Grossly incompetent Cockett's perforator, color duplex image.

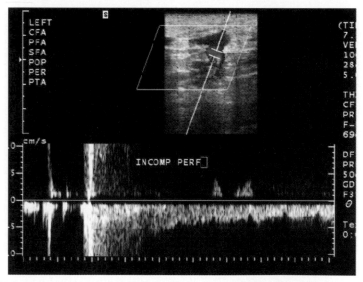

Figure 15.9 Grossly incompetent Cockett's perforator with spectral Doppler reflux signal.

appropriate reason for the use of VDU. Specific symptoms related to these conditions and situations arising for the clinician which may drive the use of VDU include limb pain of unknown etiology, tenderness to palpation of the limb, swelling or edema of the limb, varicosities, impending or current venous leg ulceration (Figures 15.12 & 15.13), and signs of clinical venous insufficiency. In addition, dyspnea, unexplained cough, or pleuritic chest pain, as possible

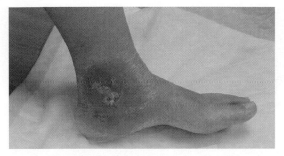

Figure 15.10 Cockett's blowout ulcer.

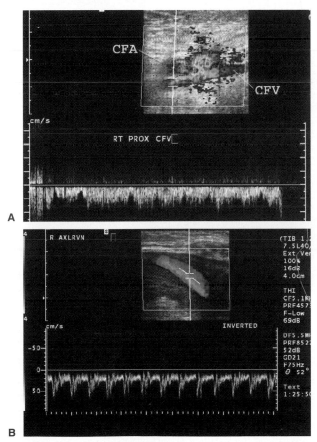

Figure 15.11 (A) Arteriovenous fistula (iatrogenic) with common femoral vein (CFV) pulsatile signal 4 days after a coronary angiogram. CFA = common femoral artery. (B) Axillary vein pulsatility on the side of a functioning arteriovenous dialysis fistula.

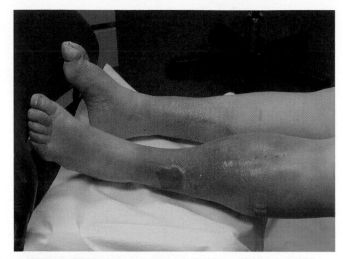

Figure 15.12 Severe chronic venous insufficiency.

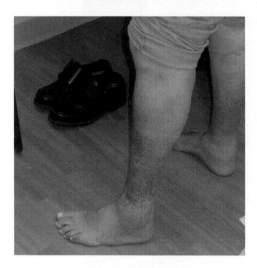

Figure 15.13 Same patient as in Figure 15.12 with severe chronic venous insufficiency after compression therapy.

symptoms of PE, may in certain situations also appropriately cause the concerned clinician to order VDU.

High-risk patient populations, such as those in the immediate post-operative period, especially following orthopedic or genito-urinary tract surgery, those with paralysis or conditions limiting mobility, including the nursing home population, high-risk inpatients with serious comorbid medical disease, such as congestive heart failure, pregnant patients, those with recent major trauma, those with morbid obesity, and those with malignancy, all pose challenging situations on a regular basis for clinicians of many specialties and in primary care. Certainly, all of these situations give rise to increased risk for VTE. "Screening" such patient populations for DVT has not, however, been identified consistently as a cost-effective method of care. A recent prospective study of 62 patients who were ambulatory, not on anticoagulants, but undergoing active chemotherapy for lung cancer and lymphoma (stage III, IV, or recurrent), and without clinical evidence of VTE, failed to find a single episode of proximal DVT in all 124 limbs[30]. This lack of prevalent thrombosis existed in this cohort even in the face of the study population having significantly higher levels of D-dimer and significantly lower levels of activated protein C ratio than controls.

Instrumentation and necessary components for laboratory output

VDU is extremely operator dependent, and the quality of the examination can vary from technologist to technologist, and from laboratory to laboratory. It is for this reason that standards for basic instrumentation and guidelines for what constitutes appropriate testing protocols exist[30]. VDU requires gray scale imaging with transverse transducer compressions and spectral Doppler evaluation with or without color imaging. A 2.5 MHz or greater duplex probe must be available for investigating the veins according to the Intersocietal Accreditation of Vascular Laboratories (ICAVL) guidelines. Practically speaking, the lower frequency probes in the 2.5–3.5 MHz frequency range are used almost exclusively for the vena cava, the iliac veins, the visceral veins, and in cases of exceptionally swollen or large limbs where penetration to view a deeply situated vein is necessary. The majority of VDU examinations of the lower and upper extremities should be performed with 5–10 MHz probes. Color Doppler has become commonly available on most new ultrasound machines and has found great applicability for use in venous scanning. Its availability has greatly improved the identification and functional imaging of calf veins in particular (Figures 15.14 & 15.15).

Without a doubt, while a good quality ultrasound unit is essential for a vascular laboratory, the technologist's knowledge base and experience to adequately

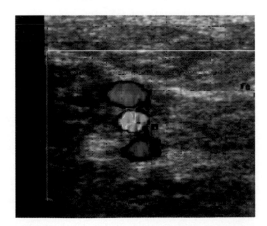

Figure 15.14 Transverse paired posterior tibial veins and artery.

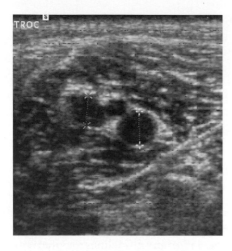

Figure 15.15 Gray scale gastrocnemius veins.

adjust the velocity range parameters and the image so as to acquire and optimize both the image and the velocity data are essential to a good quality examination and to the delivery of high-quality diagnostic information. The technologist's ability and experience are two of the most important variables facing all vascular laboratories, and these variables can make the difference between a good study and a poor study, and between a good laboratory and a poor laboratory. The acquisition of the data necessary to generate a report needs to be meticulously recorded so that a final report can be generated in a timely fashion.

The final report for all vascular laboratory studies should contain the required elements defined by accreditation standards, and should clearly indicate the identification of the patient, the date of the study, its indications, a body of data supporting the impressions (which should be clearly stated in a separate section from the body of the report), and the interpreting physician's signature.

Scanning technique and diagnostic criteria for deep vein thrombosis

The protocol for lower extremity examinations starts proximally and works distally from the common femoral vein (CFV) (Figure 15.16). The examination typically starts on the right side, beginning scanning from the CFV through the calf, and only when the right side has been completed does one proceed to the left. It is imperative that a written laboratory examination protocol (see Appendix 2), standardized for each practice and laboratory, is in place and is followed at each testing site to help guarantee uniformity in the performance of the examination across the practice regardless of technologist, machine, or testing site. Individual "styles" of performing examinations have little or no place in a well-run vascular laboratory. A key part of the technical director's and medical director's role in overseeing quality is to help ensure standardization of the examination across the practice.

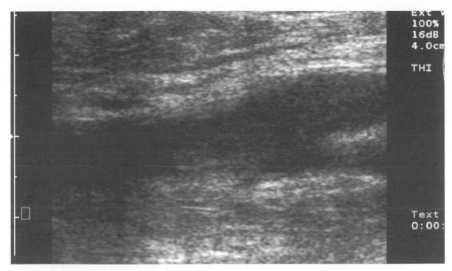

Figure 15.16 Common femoral vein with deep vein thrombosis.

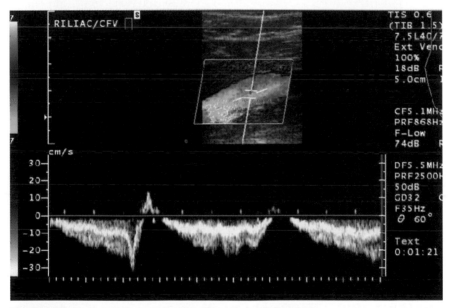

Figure 15.17 Normal respiratory phasicity of the common femoral vein.

Defining the SFJ site and demonstrating both transverse vein wall compressions and spontaneous venous Doppler signals of the CFV which are phasic with respiration are essential in establishing a normal examination (Figure 15.17). Diagnostic criteria for an abnormal examination consistent with thrombosis (Table 15.1) include a lack of or decreased spontaneity of the venous

Table 15.1 Duplex criteria for deep vein thrombosis (DVT).

Characteristic of vein	Normal	Acute DVT	Chronic DVT
Compressibility	Complete	None or minimal	Variable but > 50% unless vein contracted
Echogeneity	None unless stasis present	Hypoechoic	Hyperechoic
Diameter	Normal	Dilated	Contracted or normal
Spectral Doppler	Respirophasic and spontaneous (in proximal veins)	None or decreased with continuous flow	Variable
Response to distal augmentation	Quick upstroke and velocity	Muted or absent upstroke and velocity	Variable but usually decreased upstroke
Color Doppler	Full filling with augmentation	None or "rim pattern"	Interlaced among echogeneity

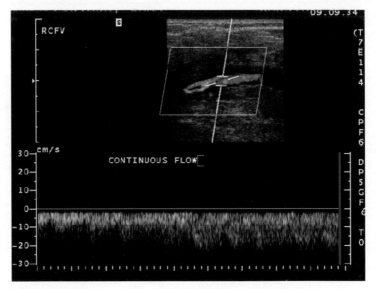

Figure 15.18 Continuous spectral venous flow; no respirophasicity.

spectral Doppler signal, lack of vein wall compression in the transverse view, and the presence of echoes in the noncompressible portion of the vein (Figures 15.18 & 15.19). Color Doppler may be used to enhance the edge of the thrombus, enhance calf vein image identification, and to help clarify whether a thrombus is totally or subtotally occluding a vein. It can also be used to demonstrate the tip of a DVT (Figure 15.20), as well as to provide evidence for a recanalized segment of thrombus (Figure 15.21). The proximal femoral vein, mid-femoral vein, and popliteal vein are examined in a similar fashion as the CFV. Vein wall compression in the transverse view in multiple sites as one progresses down the limb is essential in making certain that segmental thrombosis

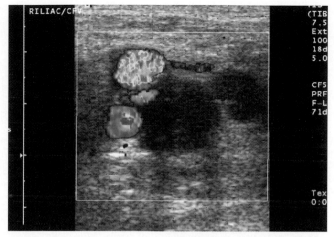

Figure 15.19 Acute common femoral vein deep vein thrombosis, transverse view.

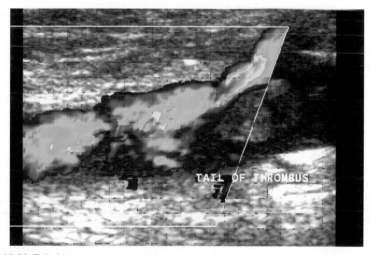

Figure 15.20 Tail of thrombus.

does not exist. Depending on the protocol in each laboratory, insonation of varying sites for spontaneity and phasicity should be performed according to accreditation standards. The distal augmentation signal (Figure 15.22) is very important in documenting patency between the site of manual compression and insonation. Repetitively attempting to augment a vein signal in a leg with a demonstrated thrombus is not advisable, however, once the diagnosis of DVT has been established.

Ever since the use of the CW Doppler technique, prior to the advent of VDU, it has been known that occlusive or near totally occlusive proximal iliac level venous thrombosis in the absence of extension of thrombus distally down to the

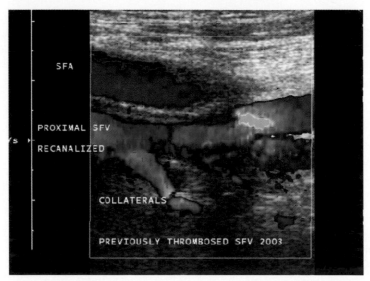

Figure 15.21 Venous collaterals.

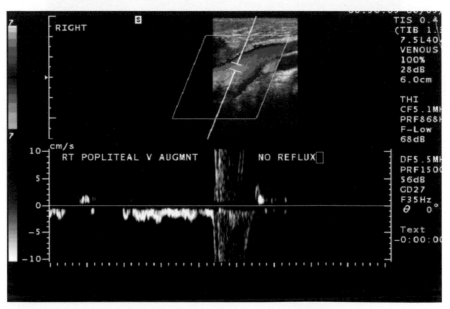

Figure 15.22 Augmentation signal indicating patency.

femoral vein (isolated iliac vein thrombus) can be discovered by an abnormal Doppler signal in a "patent" femoral vein. Such a situation will yield markedly reduced spontaneous venous flow with reduced or absent respiratory signal variations at the femoral vein level. An early case report, published in 1989 in the *New England Journal of Medicine*, demonstrated this well[31], and of all the types of clinical situation in which one does not want to see a "false negative scan," it is precisely in these instances of proximal "widow-maker" clots. Proponents of the use of infra-inguinal venous ultrasound probe compression as the sole diagnostic criterion for DVT and of doing away with spectral Doppler insonation of the proximal deep veins have long said that isolated iliac vein thrombi are relatively rare. Sarpa *et al*.[32], in 1991, showed, however, that this dangerous clinical situation, isolated iliac vein thrombosis, existed in 5% of DVTs in a series of 237 consecutive patients. However, this same prospective series indicated that duplex was only able to visualize the iliac vein directly, adequately for diagnostic purposes, in 60% of patients in the series. In my clinical experience, the current percentage of iliac veins adequately visualized by VDU, sufficient for direct diagnostic level demonstration of iliac vein thrombi, is closer to 75–80%, still significantly less than the imaging capacity of VDU for infra-inguinal leg veins.

It is precisely because of such data that ICAVL venous examination standards include the insonation of proximal femoral (CFV) venous segments with spectral Doppler, observing for spontaneity and respirophasicity of the signal. It is also for this reason that it makes good sense to insonate the contralateral CFV when performing unilateral venous scans, even when they are considered to be normal (also an ICAVL requirement), to make certain that the observed venous phasicity and spontaneity are symmetric.

It is worth noting in this world of imaging that augmentation of the spectral venous signal is a long-standing, validated, supporting data point[33] in helping to ensure vein patency, and is particularly useful in the examination of those areas of venous anatomy that are more difficult to visualize directly, such as the mid-thigh at the adductor canal level and the calf. The augmentation maneuver, best employed using a firm, distal, manual calf squeeze, also capitalizes on the observed finding that, after quickly squeezing and then rapidly releasing the calf or thigh distal to an insonated area, while "listening" with spectral Doppler at a more proximal point, a good brief augmentation of venous velocity should occur in the normal situation, regardless of the anatomic level being insonated. The absence of such augmentation, or marked muting of the velocity increase, is one key element of an abnormal examination, and should alert the technologist or the interpreting physician to look more closely at the intervening segment of vein for a possible clot. The distal augmentation maneuver is also used to generate the spectral Doppler signal from which the reflux signal is assessed when studying a patient for CVI.

In addition to venous thrombosis of the lower and upper extremities, other alternative diagnoses are often discovered in symptomatic individuals undergoing VDU. Baker's cysts (see Figure 15.23) represent one of the more common alternative diagnoses, and thrombosed popliteal artery aneurysms (see Figure 15.24) represent one of the more clinically significant "ancillary" discoveries found in the vascular laboratory during VDU. Significantly abnormal appearing lymph nodes may also occasionally be seen.

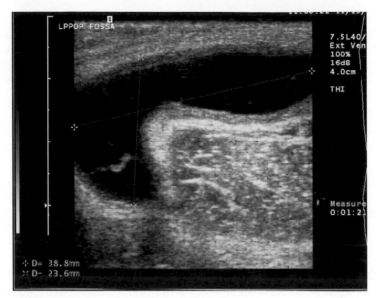

Figure 15.23 Baker's cyst.

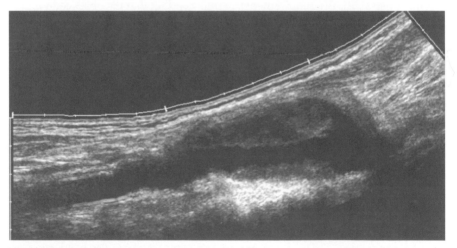

Figure 15.24 Popliteal artery aneurysm, longitudinal view.

Venous duplex ultrasonography in venous insufficiency and varicosities

In addition to DVT and PE, the other major category of patients appropriate for study with VDU are those with lower extremity venous valvular incompetence. There is a great deal of interest currently in the nonsurgical treatment of CVI, and thus a strong interest in the use of VDU to effectively assess those being considered for intervention. Because CVI is primarily caused by decreased calf pump muscle function and valvular incompetence of any one venous system (superficial, deep, or perforators) or any combination of venous systems, and because the chosen treatment regimens may be significantly different depending on which system or systems are involved, it is very important to understand the use of VDU in the assessment of CVI.

Furthermore, it has been demonstrated that DVT may not be a prerequisite for the development of both venous stasis and ulceration in up to 75% of affected limbs[34]. As Markel et al.[35] noted, up to half a million Americans may have venous ulceration, but six to seven million have stasis dermatitis and approximately 10% of the American population has varicosities. Given the prevalence and burden of venous disease in the American population, it is understandable that there is a desire to rapidly and accurately assess CVI. Because VDU has the potential to identify specific incompetent veins and their anatomic relationships to varicosities (Figure 15.25) and perforators, and to follow the results of percutaneous endovenous therapy (Figures 15.26–15.28) and simultaneously exclude DVT, it has become the test of choice for the evaluation of CVI.

Although quantitative reflux assessment using a pneumatic cuff for rapid inflation and deflation has been studied and proposed by some investigators, many vascular laboratory directors and technologists feel that it is somewhat cumbersome and time consuming to use. Quantitative and qualitative assessment of reflux can be achieved effectively by utilizing a manual compression technique of the calf with the patient in the dependent or standing position, as demonstrated in Figures 15.29 & 15.30. A prolonged reflux signal (retrograde flow) is the hallmark of venous valvular incompetence. A retrograde signal of > 0.5 s in duration is felt to represent clinical insufficiency of the superficial

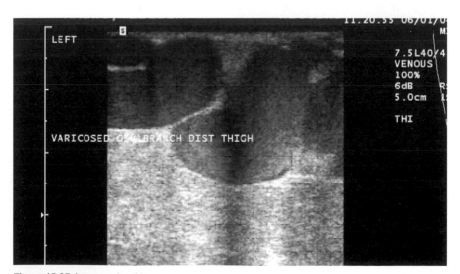

Figure 15.25 Large varicosities.

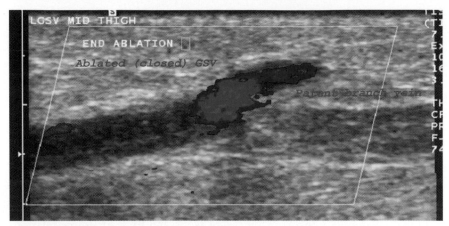

Figure 15.26 Ablated greater saphenous vein with patent branch vein.

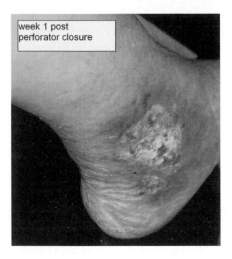

Figure 15.27 Original ulcer.

saphenous system, and a reflux signal of > 1 s in duration is felt to represent clinical deep venous insufficiency of the femoral and popliteal levels[36].

Summary

Venous disease, including DVT, PE, VTE, Vv, and CVI, is the most common form of vascular disease affecting America and maybe the world at large. From the point of view of the vascular laboratory, we are only now seeing the same level of widespread scientific interest applied to these venous diseases as has been applied for so long to the arterial diseases associated with atherosclerosis. Few technologies have had such a profound impact as duplex ultrasound in such a short period of time on how a group of closely related illnesses is assessed,

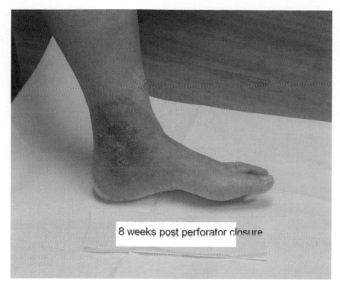

Figure 15.28 Same patient as in Figure 15.27, 8 weeks post-closure.

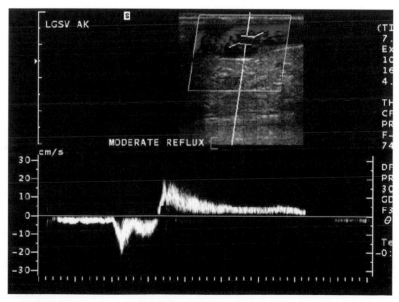

Figure 15.29 Gross reflux near saphenofemoral junction.

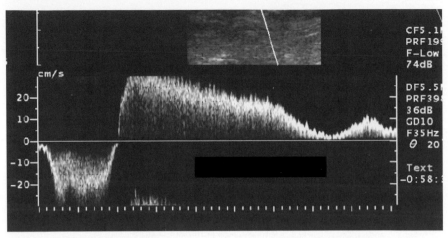

Figure 15.30 Severe reflux signal.

diagnosed, treated, and researched. It appears that VDU will continue to serve not only as an effective and readily available tool in the diagnosis of DVT and VTE, but will have an expanding role in the future in the clinical and scientific realms of CVI treatment and investigation.

Reference list

1 Coon WW, Willis PW, Keller JB. Venous thromboembolism and other venous disease in the Tecumseh community health study. Circulation 1973; 48:839–846.

2 Gillum RF. Pulmonary embolism and thrombophlebitis in the United States, 1970–1985. Am Heart J 1987; 114:1262–1264.

3 Anderson FA Jr, Wheeler HB, Goldberg RJ, et al. A population-based perspective of the hospital incidence and case-fatality rates of deep vein thrombosis and pulmonary embolism: the Worcester DVT Study. Arch Intern Med 1991; 151:933–938.

4 Nordstrom M, Lindblad B, Bergqvist D, Kjellstrom T. A prospective study of the incidence of deep-vein thrombosis within a defined urban population. J Intern Med 1992; 232:155–160.

5 Kierkegaard A. Incidence of acute deep vein thrombosis in two districts: a phlebographic study. Acta Chir Scand 1980; 146:267–269.

6 Callum MJ. Epidemiology of varicose veins. Br J Surg 1994; 81:167–173.

7 Smith JJ, Garratt AM, Guest M, Greenhalgh RM, Davies AH. Evaluating and improving health-related quality of life in patients with varicose veins. J Vasc Surg 1999; 30:10–19.

8 Kroeger K, Ose C, Rudofsky G, Roesner J, Hirche H. Risk factors for varicose veins. Intern Angiol 2004; 23:29–34.

9 Silverstein MD, Heit JA, Mohr DN, Petterson TM, O'Fallon WM, Melton LJ III. Trends in the incidence of deep vein thrombosis and pulmonary embolism: a 25-year population-based study. Arch Intern Med 1998; 158:585–593.

10 Heit JA, Silverstein MD, Mohr DN, Petterson TM, O'Fallon WM, Melton LJ III. Risk factors for deep vein thrombosis and pulmonary embolism: a population-based case–control study. Arch Intern Med 2000; 160:809–815.

11 Rabinov K, Paulin S. Roentgen diagnosis of venous thrombosis in the leg. Arch Surg 1972; 104:134–144.

12 Strandness DE Jr, Sumner DS. Ultrasonic velocity detector in the diagnosis of thrombophlebitis. Arch Surg 1972; 104:180–183.

13 Meadway J, Nicolaides AN, Walker CJ, O'Connell JD. Value of Doppler ultrasound in diagnosis of clinically suspected deep vein thrombosis. Br Med J 1975; 4:552–554.

14 Sumner DS, Lambeth A. Reliability of Doppler ultrasound in the diagnosis of acute venous thrombosis both above and below the knee. Am J Surg 1979; 138:205–210.

15 Cranley JJ, Gay AY, Grass AM, et al. Plethysmographic technique for the diagnosis of deep venous thrombosis of the lower extremities. Surg Gynecol Obstet 1973; 136:385–394.

16 Hull R, Hirsh J, Sackett DL, et al. Replacement of venography in suspected venous thrombosis by impedance plethysmography and ^{125}I-fibrinogen leg scanning: a less invasive approach. Ann Intern Med 1981; 94:12–15.

17 Hull RD, Hirsh J, Carter CJ, et al. Diagnostic efficacy of impedance plethysmography for clinically suspected deep-vein thrombosis: a randomized trial. Ann Intern Med 1985; 102:21 28.

18 Huisman MV, Buller HR, ten Cate JW, Vreeken J. Serial impedance plethysmography for suspected deep venous thrombosis in outpatients. The Amsterdam General Practitioner Study. N Engl J Med 1986; 314:823–828.

19 Huisman MV, Buller HR, ten Cate JW, Heijermans HS, van der Laan J, van Maanen DJ. Management of clinically suspected acute venous thrombosis in outpatients with serial impedance plethysmography in a community hospital setting. Arch Intern Med 1989; 149:511–513.

20 Killewich LA, Bedford GR, Beach KW, Strandness DE Jr. Diagnosis of deep venous thrombosis: a prospective study comparing duplex scanning to contrast venography. Circulation 1989; 79:810–814.

21 Lensing WA, Prandoni P, Brandjes D, et al. Detection of deep-vein thrombosis by real-time B-mode ultrasonography. N Engl J Med 1989; 320:342–345.

22 Rose SC, Zwiebel WJ, Nelson BD, et al. Symptomatic lower extremity deep venous thrombosis: accuracy, limitations, and role of color duplex flow imaging in diagnosis. Radiology 1990; 175:639–644.

23 Comerota AJ, Katz ML, Greenwald LL, et al. Venous duplex imaging: should it replace hemodynamic tests for deep venous thrombosis? J Vasc Surg 1990; 11:53–61.

24 Mitchell DC, Grasty MS, Stebbings WSL, et al. Comparison of duplex ultrasonography and venography in the diagnosis of deep venous thrombosis. Br J Surg 1991; 78:611–613.

25 Raghavendra BN, Horii SC, Hilton S, Subramanyam BR, Rosen RJ, Lam S. Deep vein thrombosis: detection by probe compression of veins. J Ultrasound Med 1986; 5:89–95.

26 Rollins DL, Semrow C, Friedell M, Calligaro K, Buchbinder D. Progress in the diagnosis of deep venous thrombosis: the efficacy of real-time B-mode ultrasonic imaging. J Vasc Surg 1988; 7(5):638–641.

27 Ricci S, Georgiev M. Ultrasound anatomy of the superficial veins of the lower limb. J Vasc Tech 2002; 26:183–199.

28 Pieri A, Gatti M, Santini M, Marcelli F, Carnemolla A. Ultrasonographic anatomy of the deep veins of the lower extremity. J Vasc Tech 2002; 26:201–211.

29 Intersocietal Accreditation Commission. ICAVL: Essentials and Standards for Accreditation in Noninvasive Vascular Testing. Part II. Vascular Laboratory Operations—Peripheral Venous Testing, 2000. www.icavl.org

30 Bernstein R, Haim N, Brenner B, Sarig G, Bar-Sela G, Gaitini D. Venous sonography for the

diagnosis of asymptomatic deep vein thrombosis in patients with cancer undergoing chemotherapy. J Ultrasound Med 2004; 23:655–658.

31 Gocke J, Harlan J. Diagnosis of isolated iliac vein thrombi by venous duplex sonography. N Engl J Med 1989; 321(9):letter 613.

32 Sarpa S, Messina L, Smith M, Chang L, Greenfield L. Reliability of venous duplex scanning to image the iliac veins and to diagnose iliac vein thrombosis in patients suspected of having acute deep venous thrombosis. J Vasc Tech 1991; 15(6):299–302.

33 Yao J, Blackburn D. Doppler venous survey. In: Kempczinski R, Yao J (eds), Practical Noninvasive Vascular Diagnosis, ch. 16, pp. 263–275. Chicago: Year Book Medical Publishers, 1982.

34 Labropoulos N, Delis K, Nicolaides AN, Leon M, Ramaswami G, Volteas N. The role of the distribution and anatomic extent of reflux in the development of signs and symptoms in chronic venous insufficiency. J Vasc Surg 1996; 23(3):504–510.

35 Markel A, Manzo R, Bergelin RO, Strandness DE. Valvular reflux after deep vein thrombosis: incidence and time of occurrence. J Vasc Surg 1992; 15(2):377–382.

36 Labropoulos N, Tiongson J, Pryor L, et al. Definition of venous reflux in lower-extremity veins. J Vasc Surg 2003; 38(4):793–798.

PART VIII

CTA and MRA of the Vascular System

16   Computerized Tomographic Angiography

Corey K. Goldman

Computerized tomographic angiography (CTA) is a rapidly advancing, noninvasive, X-ray-based modality used to image vascular anatomy rapidly and accurately. The resulting images are easily interpreted by physicians comfortable in evaluating standard contrast arteriograms (Figure 16.1). While standard computerized tomography (CT) scanning has been in the clinician's armamentarium since the mid-1970s, CTA represents a relatively new tool. Initially, standard CT scans did not provide sufficient image resolution or examination speed to be clinically useful[1]. With the advent of spiral CT and, subsequently, multidetector computerized tomography (MDCT), CTA is emerging as a useful technique for the evaluation of arterial and venous disease in clinical practice.

Several studies comparing four-detector CTA with other diagnostic modalities have indicated that CTA is both sensitive and specific for most vascular pathology in vessels with a lumen diameter of ≥ 2 mm. Clinical trials are actively comparing images obtained with newer CT scanners with those obtained by digital subtraction angiography (DSA). Many institutions are now employing CT scanners with 16 or more detectors, and the results are encouraging[2,3].

An important advantage of CTA compared with other imaging modalities (i.e. duplex ultrasonography, magnetic resonance arteriography) is the ability to depict vessels and surrounding anatomy in three dimensions. In addition, automated edge detection software allows rapid electronic measurement of lumen diameters in three-dimensional space. In contrast, digital subtraction arteriography represents a two-dimensional projection of a three-dimensional structure, increasing the likelihood of underestimation of the severity of an eccentric arterial stenosis. In theory, CTA should provide more accurate images than DSA; however, currently, there are very few anatomic studies to support this claim as DSA is considered to be the gold standard. CTA is currently being used for the evaluation of all forms of arterial disease, including atherosclerotic disease, fibromuscular dysplasia[4], dissections, aneurysms, congenital arterial abnormalities[5], and arteriovenous malformations.

As CTA represents a "snapshot" of the vessel, one limitation is that flow and direction cannot be determined. Nevertheless, CTA has already become the primary imaging modality for the initial evaluation of pulmonary embolism (PE)[6].

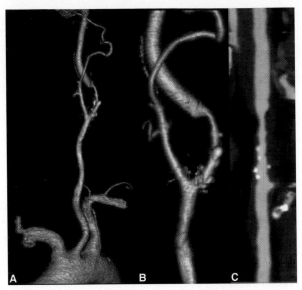

Figure 16.1 A case of carotid stenosis. The patient was referred for evaluation of asymptomatic left internal carotid artery stenosis with estimated 60–79% diameter reduction on carotid duplex ultrasonography. However, duplex examination was suboptimal because of dense calcific plaque in the carotid bulb. (A) Three-dimensional volume-rendered computerized tomographic angiography of the aortic arch, left common carotid artery, and left internal carotid artery quickly portrays the patient's anatomy. Magnification of the carotid bulb (B) allows for improved visualization of the anatomy in question. Vessel analysis was undertaken using curved multiplaner reconstruction (C) and allows for linearization of the lumen. Exact measurements could be taken from the reconstructed image.

Multidetector computerized tomography technology and technique

Early-generation CT scanners obtain discrete axial images by a circular rotation of the X-ray source and a single X-ray detector situated 180° apart on a rotating CT machine. Each subsequent image is obtained by advancing the patient gantry longitudinally in the z axis. Therefore, each image represents a discrete data set related to the next image only by its relation to the z axis. Single-detector spiral CT advances the patient gantry simultaneously with the rotation of the X-ray source and detector. Image reconstruction takes place using a continuous set of data obtained in a spiral fashion (Figure 16.2A). This allows for rapid image acquisition. By situating multiple detectors along the axial plane, multiple continuous data sets are generated and image reconstruction takes place using integration and interpolation. By switching from single-detector spiral CT to four-detector MDCT, image acquisition can take place four times faster (Figure 16.2B). Alternatively, by keeping the scanning time the same, image quality and resolution are substantially improved. Another difference between CTA and standard body CT scanning relates to image thickness. CTA obtains images 0.5–2 mm thick, while body CT obtains images 3–5 mm thick. As a result,

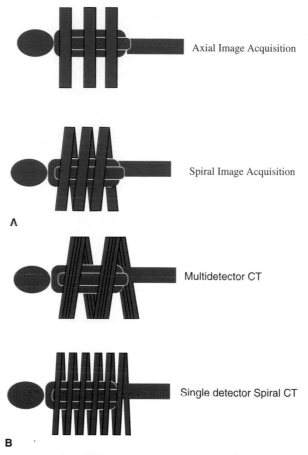

Axial Image Acquisition

Spiral Image Acquisition

Λ

Multidetector CT

Single detector Spiral CT

B

Figure 16.2 (A) Early computerized tomography (CT) scanners obtain scans using only axial image acquisition. In this mode, the X-ray source and the detector acquire images horizontally across the body. Subsequently, the X-ray source and detector rotate by a fixed angle and the planar image acquisition is begun again. Once 180° of image acquisition is complete, the gantry advances, and the next set of images is obtained. Image acquisition is acquired in discrete data sets. Spiral CT acquisition allows rotation of the X-ray source and detector, simultaneously with advancing of the patient through the X-ray beam. Spiral CT results in a continuous data set which requires a different reconstruction algorithm compared with axial image acquisition. (B) Multidetector CT scanning is commonly performed in a spiral mode. More information is obtained and a greater distance is traversed in a fixed period of time as more detectors are added. The figure compares a single-detector CT scanner with a four-detector CT scanner.

routine CTA studies will generate three or four times the number of images as routine CT studies, thereby providing a significant increase in the amount of information.

Image acquisition relative to the timing of iodinated contrast injection is central to obtaining high-quality CTA images. Ideally, image capture takes place during the first arterial pass of iodinated contrast for CT arteriography, and during peak venous opacification for CT venography. In comparison, standard body CT scanning occurs after equilibration of both phases. Some centers implement CTA scanning protocols which capture images during a noncontrast phase, an arterial phase, and a late phase. By doing so, all aspects of imaging are addressed, including the identification of bleeding sites, vascular pathology, and tissue enhancement. A major drawback is the increased radiation exposure to the patient.

Computerized tomographic angiography applications

Carotid artery disease

Images of the entire aortic arch, the great vessels, and its branches are commonly obtained in less than 1 min using MDCT. Interrogation and visualization of the carotid arteries can be performed using three-dimensional "volume" rendering or curved planar reconstruction (Figure 16.1). In clinical practice, calcified lesions poorly assessed using ultrasound (US) can often be assessed and measured using CTA (Figure 16.3). Trials examining carotid stent restenosis have not yet been published; however, there are reports confirming the use of CTA for the identification of stent restenosis in other vascular beds.

When compared with DSA, one study examining the utility of CTA for the evaluation of carotid stenosis reported a sensitivity of 95% and a specificity of 98% for the identification of significant stenosis[7]. In one series examining patients with severe near-occlusions (i.e. "string sign"), CTA demonstrated nearly 100% accuracy[8]. Despite several other single center trials confirming a high degree of accuracy, a multicenter trial (CARMEDAS) comparing CTA, magnetic resonance angiography (MRA), and US demonstrated no statistical difference in the degree of stenosis identified. However, there was greater concordance

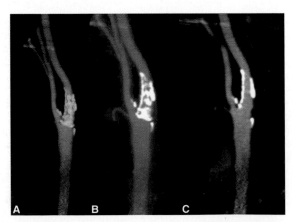

Figure 16.3 In this carotid bulb, the presence of circumferential calcium limits the utility of three-dimensional volume-rendered images (A) and maximum intensity projections (B). Using curved multiplanar reformation, computerized tomographic angiography is able to depict the vessel lumen as a thin section (C). The curved multiplanar image in (C) demonstrates a calcified carotid artery reconstructed at 1 mm thickness.

between US and contrast-enhanced MRA compared with US and CTA, and the authors suggested an inferiority for CTA. A major drawback of this trial was that > 80% of the CTA discordance came from a single institution[9].

Two studies have examined the impact of lesion eccentricity on accuracy, indicating that CTA vs. DSA concordance rates diminish as the lesion eccentricity increases. Thus, eccentric or "U-shaped" lesions may be measured as severe on CTA, but may appear as mild or moderate on DSA. In this context, US velocity information may be useful to determine whether there is a flow-limiting stenosis, especially when there is a discrepancy. At my institution, carotid lesions which represent equivocal revascularization candidates based on duplex ultrasonography, with an estimated stenosis of 60–79%, are often referred for CTA for more precise lesion characterization, although more data are needed to support this practice[10].

Vertebral artery imaging

CTA for the evaluation of the vertebral arteries or the posterior cerebral circulation produces high-quality diagnostic images[11]. Standard CTA cervical evaluation of suspected vertebrobasilar insufficiency allows for the visualization of the vertebral arteries and carotid arteries and, in some cases, may obviate the need for carotid duplex ultrasonography. Curved planar reconstructions can produce depictions of an entire cervical vertebral artery in a single image.

Several reports have suggested that CTA visualizes lesions that are poorly characterized on DSA (Figure 16.4)[12]. A recent series has confirmed the utility of CTA for imaging vertebral artery dissection[8].

Intracranial circle of Willis

Detailed evaluation of the integrity of the circle of Willis (COW) and its first-order branches is useful for the determination of collateral flow patterns in suspected transient cerebral ischemia, ischemic or hemorrhagic stroke, or subarachnoid hemorrhage. In one study, 97% sensitivity and 100% specificity were found for the identification of COW aneurysms compared with DSA[13]. For a more comprehensive brain imaging study, an initial study without contrast, followed by capture of the arterial phase for COW imaging, and finally a third run in the delayed phase can be performed. Such studies add 10–15 min to a single run study. For diagnostic purposes, electronic scrolling through planar images of the COW provides appropriate anatomic evaluation; however, three-dimensional volume reformations (Figure 16.5) often provide a complete assessment with a single view. The generation of "volume-rendered" COW images free of surrounding bone can be time consuming and requires advanced training.

Aortic imaging

Images of the aortic arch by routine body CT scanning protocols may contain movement artifact introduced by cardiac motion. The artifact is particularly relevant when evaluating ascending aortic arch dissection or aneurysms. Contem-

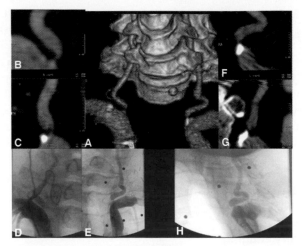

Figure 16.4 The vertebral artery origin and proximal segments can be seen using volume reconstruction after removal of adjacent mediastinal structures. (A) Severe stenosis at the origin of the right vertebral artery (left) and calcified plaque at the origin of the left vertebral artery (right). Scattered calcified plaque is also seen in the right subclavian artery. Using curved planar reconstruction, orthogonal views of the vertebral artery origins (B, C: right vertebral origin; E, F: left vertebral origin) are demonstrated and confirm bilateral vertebral artery stenosis. Digital subtraction arteriogram of the right vertebral artery in the anteroposterior plane does not convincingly reveal vertebral origin stenosis (D). Posterior inferior oblique positioning more convincingly confirms right vertebral origin stenosis (E). In this case, left vertebral origin stenosis is poorly visualized using digital subtraction angiography (H), but was confirmed using a pressure wire.

porary scanners now allow image reconstruction based on "cardiac gating," thereby allowing for freezing of mediastinal motion relative to the cardiac cycle (Figure 16.6A). By employing this method of imaging, arch images are clearer, and small dissection flaps or localized plaques can be identified (Figure 16.6B). Several studies have indicated very high sensitivity and specificity (approaching 100%) for CTA. Nonetheless, improvement in the quality of aortic arch images can be accomplished by the consideration of gating when performing CTA of the chest.

Aortic aneurysm imaging

To identify abdominal aortic aneurysms, routine body CT scanning using 3–5 mm axial section images represents a standard means of measuring aneurysm size, but is often inadequate for assessing the related mesenteric and renal arteries. In general, such studies do not allow adequate evaluations of aneurysm angulation, a key factor in determining the suitability for endovascular aortic stent-graft repair (EVAR)[14]. In contrast, CTA of the abdomen provides all of the anatomic information found in a standard CT scan, but also reveals fine vascular detail, including patency and tortuosity of the iliac arteries, aortic neck length, and angulation. The identification of renal and visceral artery orientation and patency relative to the aneurysm is also easy on standard CTA

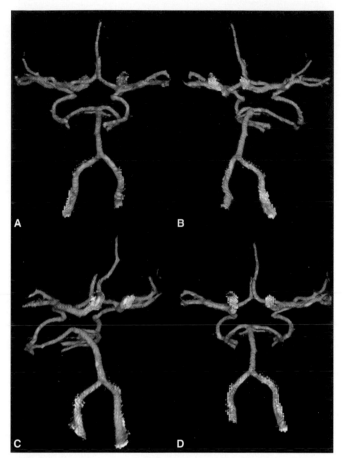

Figure 16.5 The circle of Willis is depicted in multiple views of a volume-rendered image. The circle of Willis is demonstrated in superior (A), right oblique (B), left oblique (C), and inferior (D) views. This patient does not have significant communication between the anterior and posterior circulation. Furthermore, the posterior cerebral arteries receive blood from the anterior circulation and represent an anatomic variant.

(Figure 16.6C,D). Many institutions have now replaced conventional catheter arteriography with CTA for pre-interventional evaluation. CTA has become the standard method of surveillance after EVAR, allowing for the determination of aneurysm sac regression, location and integrity of the stent-graft skeleton, and the presence of "endoleaks[14]." CTA has also been successful for the evaluation of thoracic aortic aneurysms[15] and thoracic aortic stent grafts[16].

Renal artery imaging

From a practical standpoint, CTA represents the most rapid noninvasive diagnostic test for the evaluation of the renal arteries, and can be completed in less than 10 min with minimal patient discomfort. Volume-rendered and multi-

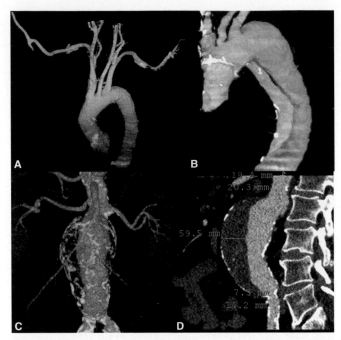

Figure 16.6 Several aspects of aortic imaging are demonstrated. (A) Three-dimensional volume-rendered image of the aortic arch and subclavian arteries. The use of cardiac gating techniques arrests cardiac-related mediastinal motion and improves aortic root imaging. When contrast is administered via an arm vein, aortic arch and great vessel images may be obscured. In (A), residual contrast can be seen along the path of the left subclavian and axillary arteries. In practice, higher magnification is used and additional reconstruction techniques are performed for diagnosis. (B) The dissection plane in this image of a Type A aortic dissection is seen as a difference in opacification intensity in the descending aortic arch. A black area demonstrates complete separation of the false and true lumen. The arrow demonstrates an aortic ring placed 10 years prior to imaging for an aortic dissection that was, at that time, limited exclusively to the ascending aorta. An abdominal aortic aneurysm is shown in (C) and (D). There is extensive thrombus in the aneurysm sac that appears transparent in the volume-rendered image (C). Calcium in the aortic wall appears as a floating rim around the aortic lumen. A sagittal planar reconstruction (D) better demonstrates the intraluminal thrombus and adjacent spine.

planar reconstructed images (Figure 16.7) are often used in conjunction for diagnosis. Although iodinated contrast is needed, isolated imaging of the abdominal aorta, including the renal arteries, can be performed using 60–80 ml of contrast[17]. The use of nonionic iso-osmolar contrast further diminishes the risk of nephrotoxicity. Renal CTA has gained rapid acceptance among renal transplant experts as an effective and noninvasive means of assessing donor kidney vascular anatomy prior to transplantation[18,19]. In my center, CTA, as a first-line screening test for renal artery stenosis (RAS), is safe, accurate, and cost-effective[20].

A meta-analysis comparing the accuracy of noninvasive modalities for the diagnosis of RAS in patients with suspected renovascular hypertension demonstrated that CTA and gadolinium-enhanced MRA had a higher diagnostic

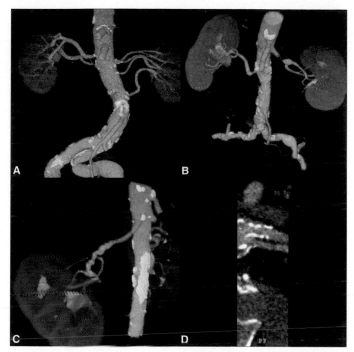

Figure 16.7 Various aspects of renal artery imaging are shown. Accessory renal arteries can be visualized easily on three-dimensional volume-rendered images (A). In this image, there is duplication of the right renal artery and triplication of the left renal artery. The right accessory renal artery (arrow) has a severe ostial stenosis. The superior left renal artery has an early bifurcation and could be misinterpreted as four left renal arteries if additional images are not examined. The left common iliac artery (*) has acute angulation. The left renal artery in (B) has a severe stenosis in the mid-distal main renal artery. This long smooth narrowing is commonly seen in association with vasculitis or the intimal hyperplasia variant of fibromuscular dysplasia. Fibromuscular dysplasia of the renal arteries can be seen on volume-rendered images (C) as well as planar images. Renal artery stents can be evaluated using planar reconstruction. In this case (D), the main renal artery (upper artery) is stented and the accessory renal artery is not stented. Both appear to be patent in this image.

accuracy than either renal artery duplex ultrasonography or nuclear scintigraphy with the administration of captopril. Willmann *et al*.[21] demonstrated 92% sensitivity and 99% specificity for four-detector CTA in the evaluation of degrees of RAS. Another study performed in 1999[22] demonstrated 94% sensitivity and 99% specificity for stenosis of > 50%. Johnson *et al*.[23] examined the various electronic reconstruction techniques for determination of the patency of renal stents, and demonstrated a sensitivity of 100% and a specificity of 97%. Comparative studies using 16-detector systems are forthcoming.

Increasingly, CTA is being performed for the evaluation of mesenteric ischemia. CTA delineates mesenteric arteries to the third or fourth branch order and also permits the evaluation of mesenteric venous thrombosis and visceral disease[20,24].

Lower extremity arterial imaging

Compared with other noninvasive diagnostic modalities (i.e. physiologic limb testing, duplex ultrasonography, magnetic resonance arteriography), CTA represents the most rapid and accurate method, often completed in 15 min. Interobserver variability is excellent, with a sensitivity and specificity near 90% or greater[25]. Post-processing can often be accomplished in 20–30 min if there is little or no calcium involving the arterial tree (Figure 16.8). However, many patients with peripheral arterial disease have extensive calcifications throughout the arterial tree, and constructing a pathway or curvilinear axis from the aorta to the infra-popliteal arteries can be time consuming. For larger arterial segments, automated pathway construction can easily be performed. For a severely calcified superficial femoral or popliteal artery, manual corrections of the automated path are often needed. In this context, thorough post-processing of an abdomen and lower extremity CTA in a patient with extensive calcification can take an hour or more. As automated post-processing programs continue to improve, more efficient programs should be forthcoming.

Several studies have demonstrated the utility and accuracy of CTA for the diagnosis of peripheral arterial disease. One study reports 99–100% sensitivity and specificity for the detection of moderate, severe, or occluded lesions[26]. In my practice, CTA of the lower extremities is useful for stratifying patients into medical, endovascular, and surgical therapeutic strategies. Not infrequently, focal symptomatic lesions have been found which were otherwise not appreciated during single view arteriography.

Imaging for restenosis

After endovascular revascularization of larger vessels with stents (i.e. iliac arteries), in-stent restenosis (intimal hyperplasia) visualization is straightforward, appearing as a dark ring between a bright stent and a bright lumen. In smaller stents, restenosis may appear eccentric or with "skip areas," which appear as darkened regions or islands adjacent to the opaque stent. The discrimination of shadow artifact from restenosis is not always possible, and some CTA studies for small vessels with stents may yield nondiagnostic information. At this time, the differentiation of restenosis from thrombus or homogeneous plaque is difficult. It is expected that in-stent imaging will improve as technology advances[27].

Venous disease

Pulmonary embolism

Spiral CT using single- or multidetector rows has become a primary tool for the diagnosis of acute PE in many centers. Although highly accurate for the identification or exclusion of central pulmonary emboli, studies comparing single-detector spiral CTA with pulmonary angiography have demonstrated diminished sensitivity in the identification of small peripheral emboli. Newer studies using MDCT have demonstrated an increased sensitivity for small peripheral emboli[28,29]. Coche et al.[29] demonstrated 96% sensitivity and 86% specificity; how-

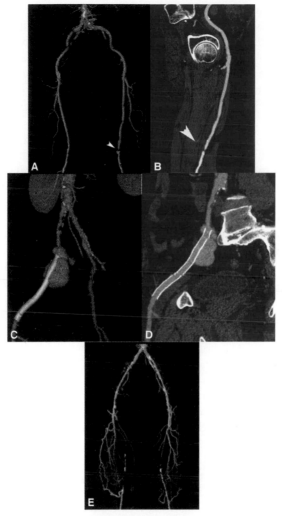

Figure 16.8 Imaging of the lower extremity arteries using computerized tomographic angiography can assist in the management of patients with peripheral arterial disease. A volume-rendered image (A) and curved multiplanar reconstruction (B) of the left superficial femoral artery both demonstrate a focal severe stenosis in a patient with lifestyle-limiting claudication. A large right external iliac artery pseudoaneurysm is demonstrated (C) in association with a long external iliac artery stent with a proximal stent fracture (D). Mild stenoses are also seen in the right common iliac artery. The patient in (E) has extensive collateralization around long bilateral superficial femoral artery occlusions. As the patient's symptoms were moderate, no invasive imaging or intervention was required.

ever, ventilation–perfusion scanning was still slightly more accurate. Kavanagh *et al.*[30] tracked 102 consecutive patients with suspected PE with negative MDCT studies. After a mean follow-up of 9 months, only one patient had a clinically important diagnosis of PE. This supports the strategy of withholding anticoagulation in patients with a negative MDCT scan.

The investigation of suspected PE with MDCT, in conjunction with D-dimer and US initially, appears to be medically sound[31]. The definitive algorithm for the diagnosis of PE remains unclear, with some suggesting that an initial ventilation–perfusion scan may be more cost-effective[32]. However, this may not be practical for some institutions. As in other vascular beds, a great advantage of CTA in the evaluation of the patient with suspected PE is that other nonvascular etiologies responsible for symptoms will be discovered (i.e. pneumonia, pneumothorax, etc.).

Deep vein thrombosis

CT venography for the evaluation of suspected large or central vein thrombosis is very useful, as it may also simultaneously reveal extrinsic compression of the culprit vein (i.e. May–Thurner anomaly)[33]. In one study, spiral CT venography for the evaluation of causes of leg swelling had a sensitivity and specificity of 100% for the identification of deep vein thrombosis, compared with US, revealing iliac vein thrombus not appreciated by ultrasonography[34]. In a similar study examining patients with known PE, CT venography was 100% sensitive and 96.6% specific for proximal deep vein thrombosis[35]. Unfortunately, there are very few studies comparing CT venography with invasive contrast venography, and therefore the utility of detecting calf vein thrombosis by CT venography is uncertain at this time.

Conclusion

The evaluation of the arterial and venous system using CTA is sensitive and specific for most vascular conditions. Compared with other noninvasive diagnostic techniques, CTA is rapid and allows for clear visualization of the surrounding anatomy. The requirement for intravenous contrast is the only significant drawback, but is often mitigated by the use of nonionic contrast and intravenous hydration. Currently, CTA technology is rapidly advancing with increased numbers of detectors, the utilization of more accurate reconstruction algorithms, and increased processor speed. While CTA has significant utility at present, the speed of technological advancement in CTA suggests even more widespread use in the future.

Reference list

1 Davis KR, Taveras JM, Roberson GH, Ackerman RH. Some limitations of computed tomography in the diagnosis of neurological diseases. Am J Roentgenol 1976; 127(1):111–123.

2 Boll DT, Lewin JS, Fleiter TR, Duerk JL, Merkle EM. Multidetector CT angiography of arterial inflow and runoff in the lower extremities: a challenge in data acquisition and evaluation. J Endovasc Ther 2004; 11(2):144–151.

3 Flohr T, Raviv-Zilka L, Cohen RA, et al. Performance evaluation of a multi-slice CT system with 16-slice detector and increased gantry rotation speed for isotropic submillimeter imaging of the heart. Herz 2003; 28(1):7–19.

4 Funabashi N, Komiyama N, Komuro I. Fibromuscular dysplasia in renovascular hypertension demonstrated by multislice CT: comparison with conventional angiogram and
   intravascular ultrasound. Heart 2003; 89(6):639.

5 Konen E, Raviv-Zilka L, Cohen RA, *et al*. Congenital pulmonary venolobar syndrome: spectrum of helical CT findings with emphasis on computerized reformatting. Radiographics
   2003; 23(5):1175 1184.

6 Remy-Jardin M, Remy J, Deschildre F, *et al*. Diagnosis of pulmonary embolism with spiral
   CT: comparison with pulmonary angiography and scintigraphy. Radiology 1996;
   200(3):699–706.

7 Hollingworth W, Nathens AB, Kanne JP, *et al*. The diagnostic accuracy of computed tomography angiography for traumatic or atherosclerotic lesions of the carotid and vertebral
   arteries: a systematic review. Eur J Radiol 2003; 48(1):88–102.

8 Chen CJ, Lee TH, Hsu HL, *et al*. Multi-slice CT angiography in diagnosing total versus near
   occlusions of the internal carotid artery: comparison with catheter angiography. Stroke
   2004; 35(1):83–85.

9 Nonent M, Serfaty JM, Nighoghossian N, *et al*. Concordance rate differences of 3 noninvasive imaging techniques to measure carotid stenosis in clinical routine practice: results of
   the CARMEDAS multicenter study. Stroke 2004; 35(3):682–686.

10 Anderson GB, Ashforth R, Steinke DE, Ferdinandy R, Findlay JM. CT angiography for the
    detection and characterization of carotid artery bifurcation disease. Stroke 2000; 31(9):
    2168–2174.

11 Sanelli PC, Tong S, Gonzalez RG, Eskey CJ. Normal variation of vertebral artery on CT
    angiography and its implications for diagnosis of acquired pathology. J Comput Assist
    Tomogr 2002; 26(3):462–470.

12 Farres MT, Grabenwoger F, Magometschnig H, Trattnig S, Heimberger K, Lammer J. Spiral
    CT angiography: study of stenoses and calcification at the origin of the vertebral artery.
    Neuroradiology 1996; 38(8):738–743.

13 Lai PH, Yang CF, Pan HB, Chen C, Ho JT, Hsu SS. Detection and assessment of circle of Willis
    aneurysms in acute subarachnoid hemorrhage with three-dimensional computed tomo-
    graphic angiography: correlation with digital subtraction angiography findings. J Formos
    Med Assoc 1999; 98(10):672–677.

14 Filis KA, Arko FR, Rubin GD, Zarins CK. Three dimensional CT evaluation for endovascu-
    lar abdominal aortic aneurysm repair. Quantitative assessment of the infrarenal aortic neck.
    Acta Chir Belg 2003; 103(1):81–86.

15 Tatli S, Yucel EK, Lipton MJ. CT and MR imaging of the thoracic aorta: current techniques
    and clinical applications. Radiol Clin North Am 2004; 42(3):565–585, vi.

16 Weigel S, Tombach B, Maintz D. Thoracic aortic stent graft: comparison of contrast-
    enhanced MR angiography and CT angiography in the follow-up: initial results. Eur
    Radiol 2003; 13(7):1628–1634.

17 Aspelin P, Aubry P, Fransson SG, Strasser R, Willenbrock R, Berg KJ. Nephrotoxic effects in
    high-risk patients undergoing angiography. N Engl J Med 2003; 348(6):491–499.

18 Urban BA, Ratner LE, Fishman EK. Three-dimensional volume-rendered CT angiography
    of the renal arteries and veins: normal anatomy, variants, and clinical applications. Radi-
    ographics 2001; 21(2):373–386; questionnaire 549–555.

19 El Fettouh HA, Herts BR, Nimeh T, *et al*. Prospective comparison of 3-dimensional volume
    rendered computerized tomography and conventional renal arteriography for surgical
    planning in patients undergoing laparoscopic donor nephrectomy. J Urol 2003; 170(1):57–60.

20 Fleischmann D. Multiple detector-row CT angiography of the renal and mesenteric vessels.
    Eur J Radiol 2003; 45(Suppl. 1):S79–S87.

21 Willmann JK, Wildermuth S, Pfammatter T, *et al*. Aortoiliac and renal arteries: prospective intraindividual comparison of contrast-enhanced three-dimensional MR angiography and multi-detector row CT angiography. Radiology 2003; 226(3):798–811.

22 Wittenberg G, Kenn W, Tschammler A, Sandstede J, Hahn D. Spiral CT angiography of renal arteries: comparison with angiography. Eur Radiol 1999; 9(3):546–551.

23 Johnson PT, Halpern EJ, Kuszyk BS, *et al*. Renal artery stenosis: CT angiography—comparison of real-time volume-rendering and maximum intensity projection algorithms. Radiology 1999; 211(2):337–343.

24 Wintersperger BJ, Nikolaou K, Becker CR. Multidetector-row CT angiography of the aorta and visceral arteries. Semin Ultrasound CT MR 2004; 25(1):25–40.

25 Martin ML, Tay KH, Flak B, *et al*. Multidetector CT angiography of the aortoiliac system and lower extremities: a prospective comparison with digital subtraction angiography. Am J Roentgenol 2003; 180(4):1085–1091.

26 Ota H, Takase K, Igarashi K, *et al*. MDCT compared with digital subtraction angiography for assessment of lower extremity arterial occlusive disease: importance of reviewing cross-sectional images. Am J Roentgenol 2004; 182(1):201–209.

27 Lawler LP, Fishman EK. Multidetector row computed tomography of the aorta and peripheral arteries. Cardiol Clin 2003; 21(4):607–629.

28 Schoepf UJ, Costello P. CT angiography for diagnosis of pulmonary embolism: state of the art. Radiology 2004; 230(2):329–337.

29 Coche E, Pawlak S, Dechambre S, Maldague B. Peripheral pulmonary arteries: identification at multi-slice spiral CT with 3D reconstruction. Eur Radiol 2003; 13(4):815–822.

30 Kavanagh EC, O'Hare A, Hargaden G, Murray JG. Risk of pulmonary embolism after negative MDCT pulmonary angiography findings. Am J Roentgenol 2004; 182(2):499–504.

31 Perrier A, Roy PM, Aujesky D, *et al*. Diagnosing pulmonary embolism in outpatients with clinical assessment, D-dimer measurement, venous ultrasound, and helical computed tomography: a multicenter management study. Am J Med 2004; 116(5):291–299.

32 Paterson DI, Schwartzman K. Strategies incorporating spiral CT for the diagnosis of acute pulmonary embolism: a cost-effectiveness analysis. Chest 2001; 119(6):1791–1800.

33 Chung JW, Yoon CJ, Jung SI, *et al*. Acute iliofemoral deep vein thrombosis: evaluation of underlying anatomic abnormalities by spiral CT venography. J Vasc Intervent Radiol 2004; 15(3):249–256.

34 Yoshida S, Akiba H, Tamakawa M, Yama N, Takeda M, Hareyama M. Spiral CT venography of the lower extremities by injection via an arm vein in patients with leg swelling. Br J Radiol 2001; 74(887):1013–1016.

35 Begemann PG, Bonacker M, Kemper J, *et al*. Evaluation of the deep venous system in patients with suspected pulmonary embolism with multi-detector CT: a prospective study in comparison to Doppler sonography. J Comput Assist Tomogr 2003; 27(3):399–409.

CHAPTER 17

17 Magnetic Resonance Imaging

Sanjay Rajagopalan

Principles of magnetic resonance angiography

Magnetic resonance angiography (MRA) can be performed with or without contrast agents. Contrast-independent techniques, such as time of flight (TOF), are dependent on the inflow of unsaturated blood (protons that have not been subjected to a radiofrequency pulse), outside the field of view, into stationary tissue within a section that is already saturated owing to its exposure to repeated radiofrequency pulses. The unsaturated blood appears bright as a consequence compared with background tissue (saturated). Contrast agent (gadolinium)-based techniques are possible because of the effects of transition metals, such as gadolinium, on the proton relaxation properties of blood, and owing to the recent refinements in gradient strengths and speeds that have allowed fast imaging within a single breath hold. This chapter briefly touches on the principles of MRA and then provides a discussion of MRA applicability in commonly encountered vascular disease states. The reader is referred to more detailed sources for a comprehensive understanding of MRA imaging[1,2].

A magnetic resonance (MR) image depends on the application of magnetic field gradients, which cause the resonant frequency of protons (the most abundant species with an unpaired electron and hence its choice in MR imaging) to vary along the axis of the magnetic field. The amplitude, phase, and frequency of MR signals are measured and used to create a map of K-space (see Glossary of special terms) that provides precise spatial and anatomic information (see Glossary of special terms). The map of K-space is then transformed to obtain an MR image (Figure 17.1)[3,4].

Paramagnetic contrast agents

Gadolinium is an element in the lanthanide transition group that exerts its effects through shortening of the T1 relaxation time of blood. This property enables the signal intensity of blood to exceed that of the surrounding content, including fat, which may appear bright on T1-weighted images[5]. The T1 shortening effect is maximized by using gadolinium chelates with high relaxivity and concentration in the blood. Generally, 0.2 mmol kg^{-1} of gadolinium is sufficient (≤ 2 bottles of 20 ml each) when performing an MR angiogram. Arteries are best imaged during the arterial phase of gadolinium infusion to take advantage of

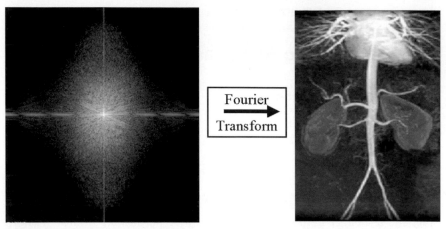

Figure 17.1 Illustration of K-space and Fourier transformation to obtain a magnetic resonance image.

the higher arterial signal-to-noise ratio (SNR) and in order to eliminate overlapping venous enhancement. A fast acquisition is essential in order to capture the contrast agent bolus during the brief moment that the agent is present in the arteries but not in the veins. This can be accomplished by a fast injection rate to ensure high concentrations in the arteries. Furthermore, differential concentrations in the arteries compared with the veins, owing to the inherent capillary extraction of gadolinium, resulting in lower venous concentration, accentuates the T1 relaxation effect in the artery compared with the vein (this effect is not present in the cerebrovascular circulation because of the blood–brain barrier and, consequently, arterial phase imaging in the central nervous system is more difficult). Phase reordering schemes that enable the acquisition of central K-space data during peak arterial gadolinium concentration, in conjunction with automated triggering schemas, allow the acquisition of high signal over spatial detail (periphery of K-space). With perfect bolus timing, high signal-to-noise arterial phase images are possible with small doses of gadolinium.

Spoiled gradient echo imaging (FLASH or SPGR)

Gradient echo sequences are the work-horse sequences for three-dimensional (3D) contrast MRA because of their speed and short echo times, which allow the acquisition of a 3D volume set in one single breath hold[6]. Spoiling helps by suppressing the background signal and thereby enhances the signal from the contrast agent in the vasculature. Additional background signal suppression, where required, can be achieved through the use of fat saturation pulses. Unlike conventional angiography, the quality of contrast MRA improves when performed rapidly. Although faster scanning is associated with a reduction in SNR related to the diminished signal averaging, there is an increase in signal intensity associated with the shorter T1 relaxation time that can be captured.

Magnetic resonance digital subtraction angiography

Image contrast can be improved by digital subtraction of pre-contrast image data from dynamic, arterial, or venous phase image data. This subtraction in MR imaging is usually performed prior to the Fourier transform using a complex subtraction method. The improvement in contrast achieved with digital subtraction angiography (DSA) may reduce the gadolinium dose required. For a good subtraction, the patient's position between the pre-contrast and contrast-enhanced images should be identical. This requirement for no motion is easily met in the pelvis and legs, but may be more difficult to achieve in the chest and abdomen, where respiratory, cardiac, and peristaltic motions are difficult to avoid. Another benefit of the subtraction is that it can be performed either on the "upslope" or "downslope" of contrast enhancement. This may result in selective visualization of arteries and veins, respectively.

Multiplanar reconstructions and maximum intensity projection

Multiplanar 3D reformations are useful in assessing the spatial relationships of vessels and to avoid vessel overlap[7,8]. Ray tracing algorithms produce maximum intensity projection (MIP) images. The maximum intensity encountered along any predefined direction is assigned to the designated pixel. The advantage of MIP images is the similarity to conventional angiographic images, which can be interpreted by most vascular physicians. Multiplanar reconstructions (MPRs) represent reconstructions that average pixel intensity across multiple overlapping planes to provide an image along a specified plane. The limitations of these reconstructed images should be understood. MIPs are well known to exaggerate stenosis, or may even artificially create a stenosis where none exists if insufficient data are available along a plane. For this reason, the estimation of stenosis severity should always be obtained from the source images.

Phase contrast magnetic resonance angiography

This technique is based on the principle that the net phase gain of flowing blood through a magnetic field gradient is proportional to its velocity. Therefore, if the phase can be derived at any point in time, the velocity can be calculated. This is accomplished by the use of a bipolar gradient and is referred to as flow encoding. Because the two bipolar gradients have equal area, stationary tissue does not incur a phase shift, while flowing blood will acquire a shift in phase that is proportional to its velocity. The resultant phase information is then reconstructed and provides a phase map of the area of interest. The phase map is then converted to a velocity map from which it is possible to derive information such as the peak velocity, mean velocity, and flow[9,10]. Phase contrast MRA (PC-MRA) can be 2D or 3D (a volume).

Magnetic resonance angiography in the diagnosis of vascular diseases

Table 17.1 lists the common MR protocols utilized when imaging specific vascu-

Table 17.1 Common protocols for anatomic areas of interest.

Thoracic aorta	Lower extremity	Renal arteries and abdominal aorta	Aortic arch and carotids
1. Localizers	1. Localizers	1. Localizers	1. Localizers
2. Axial, coronal, and sagittal dark blood sequences	2. Coronal 3D CE-MRA in 3–4 stations	2. Axial, coronal, and sagittal dark blood sequences with fat sat	2. Axial, coronal, and sagittal dark blood sequences
3. Axial and sagittal bright blood	3. 2D MR DSA of infra-popliteal vessels	3. Coronal 3D CE-MRA	3. Axial bright blood
4. Sagittal 3D CE-MRA		4. Delayed venous phase	4. When evaluating intracranial vessels — MOTSA
		5. Axial T2-weighted images	
		6. Axial 3D PC-MRA	

2D/3D = two/three-dimensional; CE-MRA = contrast-enhanced magnetic resonance angiography; DSA = digital subtraction angiography; fat sat = fat saturation pulses; MOTSA = multiple overlapping thin slab acquisition; this is an MRA technique combining the advantages of 2D and 3D time-of-flight techniques; MR = magnetic resonance; PC-MRA = phase contrast magnetic resonance angiography.

lar beds. Often concomitant anatomic images are obtained to assess morphology prior to and sometimes after (as in delayed venogram phases in renal artery imaging to assess the collecting system) contrast MRA examinations.

Three-dimensional, gadolinium-enhanced magnetic resonance angiography of the thoracic aorta

Indications
MR evaluation of the thoracic aorta provides superb delineation of the aorta. In addition to anatomic information, MRA is particularly helpful for the assessment of the physiologic significance of stenosis involving the great vessels or vertebrals, vessel flow (directionality and velocity), and thrombus. These abilities establish the role of MR as an ideal tool for the comprehensive assessment of aortic dissection and other complex aortic pathology[11].

Technique
The evaluation of the thoracic aorta begins with sequences designed to provide anatomic information. These may involve nonbreath hold, dark blood, spin echo sequences in axial, sagittal, and coronal sections. Cine sequences of the heart may be performed either before or after these in order to assess concomitant aortic valve involvement. This is followed by breath hold, electrocardiogram (EKG)-gated, gadolinium-based MRA utilizing an automated bolus tracking system, such as Smartprep (GE Medical Systems) or Care Bolus (Siemens Medical Systems). Non-EKG-gated examinations may suffice for evaluation involving the descending thoracic aorta, where movement related to

cardiac systole is less of an issue, or in instances where breath hold examinations cannot be performed owing to patient inability. Following the contrast MRA, additional sequences specific to the clinical question may be performed, e.g. PC-MRA in cases of dissection to assess flow in a false lumen or delayed enhancement imaging to assess the presence of thrombus. Assessment for inflammatory involvement of the arch and the great vessels may require additional post-gadolinium, delayed, T1-weighted, EKG-gated spin echo sequences in the axial plane with fat saturation[12].

Interpretation

The anatomic images provide gross information and cannot be relied on for specific vessel wall-related questions. Gadolinium contrast MRA images (Figure 17.2) are assessed after subtraction from mask images on a workstation. MIP and MPR images are created and the aorta and its vessels assessed in multiple planes. Subtraction of background tissue signal improves the fidelity of MIP reconstructions, especially in the regions of stenosis. In addition to the MIP images, the source images are reformatted at different angles. With active aortitis, the aortic wall is often bright on T2- and on post-gadolinium, T1-weighted images. Phase contrast imaging may reveal flow in a false lumen and is useful to assess for persistent flow in follow-up evaluations of chronic dissection[13]. Thrombus appears dark on delayed enhancement inversion recovery sequences set to a prolonged inversion time (TI).

Magnetic resonance angiography for the diagnosis of peripheral arterial disease

Indications

At many institutions, contrast MRA has replaced X-ray angiography for the diagnosis of peripheral arterial disease, except when the latter is being performed prior to a planned intervention to confirm findings. A number of studies have compared MRA with conventional angiography, and have reported sensitivities and specificities of > 90% in the diagnosis of aorto-iliac and superficial femoral arterial disease[14]. The diagnosis of infra-popliteal disease, when performed as a separate station, provides excellent resolution of vessels all the way to the foot[15]. Contrast MRA provides very good resolution of graft disease.

Technique

Contrast (gadolinium) MRA examinations are almost exclusively used in the MR evaluation of peripheral arterial disease, as TOF imaging is time consuming (may take more than 5 min to scan the aorto-iliac vessels alone) and impractical in a busy clinical service. The main difficulty in lower extremity imaging involves imaging over a very large field of view. The large field of view of the extremities is usually covered in three or four minimally overlapping imaging stations (pelvis, thigh, and leg stations). The introduction of moving tables (floating tables) has facilitated "bolus chase" 3D contrast MRA approaches,

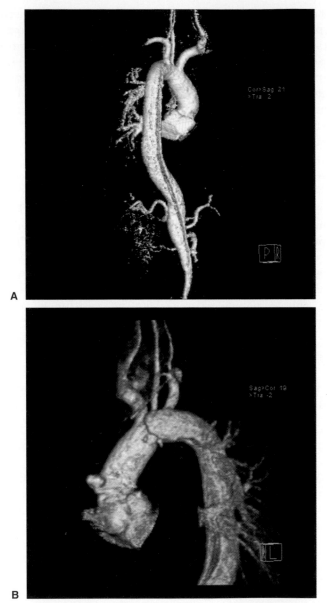

Figure 17.2 Chronic Type B dissection visualized on contrast magnetic resonance angiography of the thoracic aorta performed in a single breath hold.

where a bolus of contrast is followed down to the foot[16]. The contrast may be injected continuously or in separate boluses for each station, and the table is controlled either manually or automatically. In general, the bolus chase approach works extremely well to the level of the popliteal arteries (pelvis and thigh stations). For the visualization of vessels below the level of the popliteal artery, a separate station may also be performed prior to the bolus chase part of the examination. This may be performed using time-resolved imaging on contrast kinetics (TRICKS) (see below) or 2D MRDSA, employing local coils (head coil, extremity coil). Dynamic 2D MRDSA is ideally suited as it provides a time-resolved examination identical to an angiogram and information on the filling characteristics of distal vessels that surgeons find appealing to make bypass decisions. In addition, it provides information on bolus timing for the bolus chase part of the examination.

Three-dimensional time-resolved imaging on contrast kinetics
3D TRICKS is a scheme to increase frame rates up to 1 s per 3D volume, and relies on a number of post-processing algorithms that facilitate rapid acquisition of data within a single breath hold (more frequent sampling of central K-space, zero filling, and temporal interpolation of data). It appears to offer better resolution than conventional bolus chase techniques that do not incorporate 2D MRDSA for the visualization of infra-popliteal vessels[17,18].

Interpretation
The gadolinium-based images are subtracted from mask images and examined in multiple planes on a workstation. The pelvis, thigh, and leg stations are examined individually, and the source images are evaluated together with MIP reconstructions[19].

Magnetic resonance angiography for the diagnosis of renovascular disease

Indications
MRA is emerging as the initial examination of choice in patients with suspected renal artery stenosis[20]. Renal MRA provides anatomic and physiologic information on the severity of renal artery stenosis, besides providing additional information on neoplastic renal or abdominal masses, and ureteric anatomic information that may be relevant for the evaluation of potential renal transplant donors.

Technique
3D dynamic spoiled gradient echo imaging of the renal arteries is performed with breath hold in the coronal plane[2,21,22]. The sequence is usually repeated three times: pre-contrast, during the arterial phase, and during the venous or equilibrium phase of contrast administration (delayed images for collecting system visualization). Based on the patient's breath holding capacity, the scan time can be adjusted via the number of slices, thickness, and phase encode steps. An automated system, such as Smartprep (GE Medical Systems) or Care Bolus (Siemens Medical Systems), is used to time the gadolinium to ensure imaging during peak contrast in the renal arteries. The 3D data set is digitally subtracted from the pre-contrast mask images to obtain contrast MRA images.

Table 17.2 Interpretation of the significance of renal artery stenosis using information on three-dimensional (3D) gadolinium contrast magnetic resonance angiography (MRA) and phase contrast magnetic resonance techniques.

Grade of stenosis	3D contrast MRA findings	3D phase contrast findings
No stenosis	Normal signal	Normal signal
Mild	Stenosis is seen	Normal signal
Moderate	Stenosis is seen	± Dephasing
Severe	Stenosis	Dephasing
Occluded	Image quality good but cannot find the renal artery	No signal

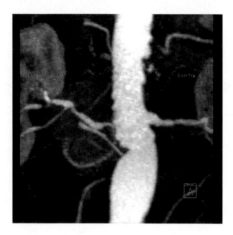

Figure 17.3 Bilateral renal artery stenosis visualized on contrast magnetic resonance angiography performed in a single breath hold. A severe proximal lesion is seen on the right renal artery and a moderate lesion in the mid-portion of the left renal artery. Note should be made of severe ulcerations in the supra-renal portion of the abdominal aorta and a small infra-renal abdominal aortic aneurysm.

Axial, three-dimensional, phase contrast magnetic resonance angiography

This sequence aids in the evaluation of the hemodynamic significance of renal artery stenosis. Performance of the sequence after gadolinium contrast imaging takes advantage of the extra signal to noise produced by the contrast agent. Once the images have been acquired, they are transferred to a workstation and post-processed with the construction of MIP and MPR.

Interpretation

The severity of renal artery stenosis is decided initially on the basis of 3D gadolinium MRA images viewed on multiple planes. This is then further evaluated on 3D phase contrast images by the presence of signal "dephasing" (Table 17.2)[2,20,22]. Normal renal artery caliber on 3D phase contrast imaging indicates normal renal arteries or, at most, mild renal artery stenosis. Severe signal "dephasing" is evidence of hemodynamically significant renal artery stenosis[23]. If the stenosis is apparent on both 3D gadolinium MRA and 3D phase contrast imaging (Figure 17.3), but there is no dephasing, it is graded as moderate. Post-stenotic dilation, loss of cortical medullary differentiation, delayed renal enhancement, and asymmetric concentration of gadolinium in the collecting system during the equilibrium phase are additional signs of hemodynamic significance.

Magnetic resonance angiography for the diagnosis of extracranial carotid and arch disease

Indications

Gadolinium-based MRA has provided a viable alternative to catheter-based angiography, which is associated with risks, and in a number or centers is performed in lieu of the latter investigation. As duplex carotid ultrasonography provides good sensitivity and specificity for high-grade carotid lesions, carotid MRA cannot be recommended routinely in every patient[24]. The current indications for carotid MRA include: (i) the assessment of disease in patients with marked vessel calcification, tortuosity, high carotid bifurcation, or other reasons that may preclude an adequate duplex evaluation; (ii) the assessment of contralateral and intracranial disease; (iii) the assessment of aortic arch disease and vertebral artery disease; and (iv) the assessment of patients with unusual presentation, particularly those with vasculitis. The advantages of gadolinium-enhanced MRA for carotid angiography include the short imaging times with excellent SNR (coverage from aortic arch to circle of Willis with a single breath hold), the ability to image ulcerations and vessel wall involvement[12,25] (in cases with vasculitis), and the inherent nonsusceptibility to flow-related artifacts.

Technique

3D contrast MRA is usually obtained in the coronal plane with triggering with an automated bolus tracking protocol (see above)[26]. The arteriovenous transit time in the cerebral circulation is extremely rapid, necessitating split second timing. The acquisition is performed with true centric K-space weighting to avoid jugular venous enhancement. Alternatively, a multiphase acquisition using the 3D TRICKS technique (3D frame rate of 3–4 s^{-1}), which results in a time-resolved examination, may be employed[27]. The short acquisition time will ensure that at least one of the volumes includes the arterial phase[28]. With time-resolved acquisition, however, there may be some compromise in spatial resolution. Breath holding improves the sharpness of the aortic arch and great vessel origins, but has no effect on the visualization of the carotid vessels. Breath holding also runs the risk of arching the neck, which moves the carotid arteries anteriorly and potentially out of the coronal imaging volume.

Interpretation

The subtracted 3D MRA images are viewed on separate workstations. Findings on MIP reconstructions should be confirmed on source images. Artifacts that are relevant to imaging the aortic arch and subclavian disease are the coil dropout artifact and the venous susceptibility artifact (see below). The former occurs in patients with a low aortic arch or elevated shoulders. The coil sensitivity of a chest coil (often used to image the aortic arch and the proximal great vessels) may drop out in the periphery, resulting in the loss of signal and simulation of a stenosis. Venous susceptibility artifact may occur around the subclavian and innominate vessels because of high concentrations of contrast agent in the venous system that may obscure the signal in the adjoining arteries. To avoid this artifact, right-hand injection is preferred, as the region of the left innominate vein is more prone to obscure the arch vessels.

Limitations

There are a large number of artifacts that can degrade data and influence findings on MRA. A knowledge of common artifacts is important in the evaluation of MR angiograms.

Susceptibility artifacts

These are effects due to the presence of metal (surgical clips, shrapnel, and stents), a high concentration of intravenous contrast agents (such as in the veins, which may interfere with arterial contrast presence), and air–tissue interfaces (such as lung–vessel or bowel–vessel interfaces). These produce focal signal dropout (dark areas in the image) that can obscure image details, decrease the visualization of surrounding vessels, and simulate stenoses or obstructions. This artifact can be minimized (but not eliminated) using imaging sequences with very short echo times (< 3 ms). The use of plain films may be required to assess the presence and location of metallic foreign bodies in the patient.

Motion artifacts

Image reconstruction algorithms in MR imaging assume stationary tissue. If there is gross body motion by an uncooperative patient, or breathing motion, the resulting images are degraded and blurred. These artifacts can be minimized by breath holding during the examination and shorter acquisition times. However, motion related to peristalsis or the pulsatility of vessels cannot be readily controlled and may cause artifacts. Intraluminal turbulence due to a stenosis may cause spin dephasing, resulting in the overestimation of stenosis.

Coverage artifacts

If parts of the vessels are not included in the acquired images, they appear as occluded vessels on MIP images. This happens, for example, in patients with a tortuous aorta. Localizing processes must be conducted carefully with the examination of pre-contrast images to confirm inclusion of the complete anatomy of interest. Vessels included near the edges of the field of view can show signal dropoff, as the coil sensitivity drops off near the edges of the coil.

Timing artifacts

Timing of the contrast bolus is of paramount importance in contrast-enhanced MRA. If the imaging is performed too early, the vessels are not sufficiently enhanced and could seem to be obstructed as a result of a low signal. This is especially important distal to a stenosis or an occlusion, when delays must be used to show all collaterals and the reconstituted vessel distal to the occlusion. Several delayed acquisitions may be necessary for complete imaging of the vessels in the case of stenosis or occlusion. Alternatively, time-resolved, dynamic, contrast-enhanced MRA or slow infusions of contrast can be performed until all the vessels of interest have filled with contrast. If the peak concentration of the bolus has not been reached during acquisition of the central portion of K-space and the T1 value of arterial blood is still changing during imaging, a ringing artifact with intraluminal, dark, longitudinal stripes of signal can mimic a dissection[29]. If the bolus is too short to cover the acquisition of the high-frequency lines in K-space, image resolution is decreased. If imaging is performed too late (most common artifact), there is contrast present in the veins during acquisition of the central part of K-space, and thus venous contamination of the images, making the results more difficult to interpret on post-processed images such as MIPs. This is especially true in the renal arteries and the carotid arteries, because of the short arteriovenous transit times.

Resolution artifacts

Limited spatial resolution limits the sensitivity to detect small lesions, such as intraluminal defects, small stenoses in vasculitis and atherosclerotic disease, small aneurysms in vasculitis, or even small vessels altogether, such as the inferior mesenteric artery. In vessels beyond the resolution of the examination, indirect findings, such as bowel mucosal enhancement on delayed images, can be used to evaluate local perfusion. "Partial voluming" as a result of thick slices can give the appearance of stenosis. If possible, imaging should be performed on multiple planes to confirm findings.

Safety checks and contraindications

Table 17.3 demonstrates a rough safety check for the assessment of the MR compatibility of metallic objects prior to undergoing an MR scan. MR imaging is contraindicated in the presence of the items listed in Table 17.3 under absolute contraindications. The reader is referred to more comprehensive sources for additional details[30].

Table 17.3 Magnetic resonance (MR) compatibility of metallic objects prior to undergoing an MR scan.

Absolute contraindications	No contraindications
Pacemakers and AICDs	Vascular stents, coils, and filter devices
Brain aneurysm clips	Vascular access clips
Metal fragments in eye	Dental devices and materials
Cochlear implants	Orthopedic metal
	Heart valves

AICD = automatic implantable cardioverter defibrillator.

Glossary of special terms

Dephasing: Disintegration of magnetization due to loss of phase coherence.

K-space: A data set that contains spatial and imaging information about an object that has been imaged. This data set is obtained by complex Fourier transformation of an original data set, and is typified by having low-frequency data in the center of K-space (dominates image contrast) and high spatial frequency in the periphery (dominates spatial detail). Contrast MRA takes advantage of this and preferentially acquires center of K-space data during the arterial phase.

Partial voluming: Intrinsic to all imaging modalities with finite limits of spatial resolution. The signals from different tissues with different signal intensities are averaged and depicted as an intermediate signal intensity.

Pulse sequences: The program that instructs the MR scanner on how to administer radiofrequency pulses at the appropriate frequency and duration, and how to balance magnetic field gradients to image the appropriate anatomic structure.

T1 relaxation: Longitudinal or spin lattice relaxation time. The time constant for spins to re-align themselves with an external magnetic field after being subjected to a perturbation. It is an intrinsic property of tissue at a given magnetic field strength. Tissues that contain water generally have longer T1 relaxation times than tissues that have abundant intracellular surface area or contain paramagnetic particles.

T2 relaxation: Otherwise referred to as the spin–spin relaxation time, this characterizes the decay characteristics of the transverse magnetization (the transverse magnetization describes the magnetization after it has been tipped into the transverse plane by a radiofrequency pulse). Initially, the spins are in phase at time zero, but gradually lose their coherence. The time constant that describes this decay is distinct from the recovery of the longitudinal relaxation, and is referred to as T2 relaxation.

TE—echo time: The time between the middle of an exciting radiofrequency pulse and the peak of the spin or gradient echo.

Time-of-flight (TOF) imaging: TOF imaging is based on the concept that "unsaturated" blood flowing into an area that has been saturated with repeated saturation pulses (thus appearing dark) will appear bright and can be distinguished from surrounding tissue. Thus the "time" it takes for the flight of blood into an image section is the mechanism for vascular enhancement. This is thus a pulse sequence that makes use of the inherent contrast of flowing blood.

TR—repetition time: The time period between the beginning of a pulse sequence and the beginning of the succeeding pulse sequence.

Reference list

1 Rajagopalan S, Prince M. Magnetic resonance angiographic techniques for the diagnosis of arterial disease. Cardiol Clin 2002; 20:501–512, v.

2 Prince MR, Grist TM, Debatin JF. 3D Contrast MR Angiography, 1st edn. Berlin: Springer-Verlag, 1999.

3 Sinha U, Sinha S, Lufkin RB. Magnetic Resonance Image Formation, 2nd edn. St. Louis, MO: Mosby-Year Book, 1997.

4 Paschal CB, Morris HD. K-space in the clinic. J Magn Reson Imaging 2004; 19:145–159.

5 Runge VM, Nelson KL. Contrast agents. In: Stark DD, Bradley JWG (eds), Magnetic Resonance Imaging, pp. 257–290. St. Louis, MO: Mosby, 1999.

6 Mitchell DG. MRI Principles, 1st edn. Philadelphia, PA: W. B. Saunders, 1999.

7 Davis CP, Hany TF, Wildermuth S, Schmidt M, Debatin JF. Postprocessing techniques for gadolinium-enhanced three-dimensional MR angiography. Radiographics 1997; 17:1061–1077.

8 Prokop M, Shin HO, Schanz A, Schaefer-Prokop CM. Use of maximum intensity projections in CT angiography: a basic review. Radiographics 1997; 17:433–451.

9 Dumoulin CL. Phase contrast MR angiography techniques. Magn Reson Imaging Clin N Am 1995; 3:399–411.

10 Pelc NJ. Flow quantification and analysis methods. Magn Reson Imaging Clin N Am 1995; 3:413–424.

11 Carr JC, Finn JP. MR imaging of the thoracic aorta. Magn Reson Imaging Clin N Am 2003; 11:135–148.

12 Atalay MK, Bluemke DA. Magnetic resonance imaging of large vessel vasculitis. Curr Opin Rheumatol 2001; 13:41–47.

13 Kunz RP, Oberholzer K, Kuroczynski W, et al. Assessment of chronic aortic dissection: contribution of different ECG-gated breath-hold MRI techniques. Am J Roentgenol 2004; 182:1319–1326.

14 Koelemay MJ, Lijmer JG, Stoker J, Legemate DA, Bossuyt PM. Magnetic resonance angiography for the evaluation of lower extremity arterial disease: a meta-analysis. J Am Med Assoc 2001; 285:1338–1345.

15 Wang Y, Winchester PA, Khilnani NM, et al. Contrast-enhanced peripheral MR angiography from the abdominal aorta to the pedal arteries: combined dynamic two-dimensional and bolus-chase three-dimensional acquisitions. Invest Radiol 2001; 36:170–177.

16 Ho VB, Corse WR. MR angiography of the abdominal aorta and peripheral vessels. Radiol Clin North Am 2003; 41:115–144.

17 Hany TF, Carroll TJ, Omary RA, et al. Aorta and runoff vessels: single-injection MR angiography with automated table movement compared with multiinjection time-resolved MR angiography—initial results. Radiology 2001; 221:266–272.

18 Swan JS, Carroll TJ, Kennell TW, et al. Time-resolved three-dimensional contrast-enhanced MR angiography of the peripheral vessels. Radiology 2002; 225:43–52.

19 Tatli S, Lipton MJ, Davison BD, Skorstad RB, Yucel EK. From the RSNA refresher courses: MR imaging of aortic and peripheral vascular disease. Radiographics 2003; 23(Spec No):S59–S78.

20 Schoenberg SO, Rieger J, Nittka M, Dietrich O, Johannson LO, Reiser MF. Renal MR angiography: current debates and developments in imaging of renal artery stenosis. Semin Ultrasound CT MR 2003; 24:255–267.

21 Schoenberg SO, Prince MR, Knopp MV, Allenberg JR. Renal MR angiography. Magn Reson Imaging Clin N Am 1998; 6:351–370.

22 Prince MR. Renal MR angiography: a comprehensive approach. J Magn Reson Imaging 1998; 8:511–516.

23 Prince MR, Schoenberg SO, Ward JS, Londy FJ, Wakefield TW, Stanley JC. Hemodynamically significant atherosclerotic renal artery stenosis: MR angiographic features. Radiology 1997; 205:128–136.

24 Back MR, Rogers GA, Wilson JS, Johnson BL, Shames ML, Bandyk DF. Magnetic resonance angiography minimizes need for arteriography after inadequate carotid duplex ultrasound scanning. J Vasc Surg 2003; 38:422–430, discussion 431.

25 Corti R, Fayad ZA, Fuster V, *et al*. Effects of lipid-lowering by simvastatin on human atherosclerotic lesions: a longitudinal study by high-resolution, noninvasive magnetic resonance imaging. Circulation 2001; 104:249–252.

26 Jewells V, Castillo M. MR angiography of the extracranial circulation. Magn Reson Imaging Clin N Am 2003; 11:585–597, vi.

27 Turski PA, Korosec FR, Carroll TJ, Willig DS, Grist TM, Mistretta CA. Contrast-enhanced magnetic resonance angiography of the carotid bifurcation using the time-resolved imaging of contrast kinetics (TRICKS) technique. Top Magn Reson Imaging 2001; 12:175–181.

28 Carroll TJ, Korosec FR, Petermann GM, Grist TM, Turski PA. Carotid bifurcation: evaluation of time-resolved three-dimensional contrast-enhanced MR angiography. Radiology 2001; 220:525–532.

29 Maki JH, Prince MR, Londy FJ, Chenevert TL. The effects of time varying intravascular signal intensity and k-space acquisition order on three-dimensional MR angiography image quality. J Magn Reson Imaging 1996; 6:642–651.

30 Shellock FG, Kanal E. Magnetic Resonance: Bioeffects and Safety. St. Louis, MO: Mosby, 1998.

Appendix 1: Appropriate ICD-9 Codes for Vascular Laboratory Tests

Carotid duplex [CPT 93880, 92882]		*Arterial duplex [lower extremity 93925 (bilateral) and 93926 (unilateral), upper extremity 93930 (bilateral) and 93931 (unilateral)] and PVR [at rest only 93923, with exercise 93924, ABI 93922 I]*	
ICD-9	*Description*	*ICD-9*	*Description*
342.00–342.92	Hemiplegia and hemiparesis	440.0	Atherosclerosis of aorta
344.00–344.9	Other-paralytic syndromes	440.21–440.24	Athero. of native
362.30–362.37	Retinal vascular occlusion		arteries/extremities
362.84	Retinal ischemia	440.21	Athero. of native
368.10	Subjective visual disturbance		arteries/ext./claud.
	unspecified	440.22	Athero. of native
368.11	Sudden visual loss		arteries/ext./rest pain
368.12	Transient visual loss	440.23	Athero. of native
368.40–368.47	Visual field defects		arteries/ext./ulceration
433.0–433.91	Occlusion and stenosis of	440.24	Athero. of native
	precerebral arteries		arteries/ext./gangrene
433.1*	Occlusion and stenosis of	440.30 440.32	Athero. of bypass graft of
	carotid		extremities
433.2*	Occlusion and stenosis of	440.30	Athero. of bypass graft of
	vertebral		ext./unspec. graft
433.3*	Occlusion and stenosis of	440.31	Athero. of bypass graft of
	multiple (bilateral)		ext/auto. vein
434.00–434.91	Occlusion of cerebral arteries	440.32	Athero. of bypass graft of
434.11	Cerebral embolism		ext/nonauto. vein
435.00–435.9	Transient cerebral ischemia	441.00–441.9	Aortic aneurysm and
435.0	Vertebral syndrome		dissection
435.1	Basilar syndrome	441.01	Dissecting thoracic aortic
435.2	Subclavian steal		aneurysm
435.9	TIA	441.02	Dissecting abdominal aortic
436	CVA; acute, ill-defined,		aneurysm
	cerebrovascular disease	441.03	Dissecting thoracoabdominal
437.0	Cerebral atherosclerosis		AA
437.3	Cerebral aneurysm,	441.2	Thoracic aortic aneurysm
	nonruptured	441.4	Abdominal aortic aneurysm
437.4	Cerebral arteritis	442.0	Other aneurysm of
437.7	Transient global ischemia		artery/upper extremity

Carotid duplex [CPT 93880, 92882]		Arterial duplex [lower extremity 93925 (bilateral) and 93926 (unilateral), upper extremity 93930 (bilateral) and 93931 (unilateral)] and PVR [at rest only 93923, with exercise 93924, ABI 93922]]	
ICD-9	Description	ICD-9	Description
442.81	Aneurysm, artery of neck	442.3	Other aneurysm of artery/lower ext./femoral
442.82	Aneurysm, subclavian artery		
446.0–446.7	Polyarteritis nodosa and allied conditions	443.0–443.9	Other peripheral vascular disease
446.5	Giant cell arteritis	443.0	Raynaud's disease
446.6	Takayasu's disease	443.9	Peripheral vascular disease;
780.2	Syncope		unspec.
780.3	Dizziness and giddiness (not payable alone)	444.0–444.9	Arterial embolism and thrombosis
781.2	Abnormality of gait	444.22	Embolism, lower extremity
781.3	Lack of coordination	447.0	Arteriovenous fistula, acquired
781.4	Transient paralysis of limb	447.1	Stricture of artery
782.0	Disturbance of skin sensation	447.2	Rupture of artery
		707.1	Ulcer of skin of lower ext.; except decubitus
784.3	Aphasia		
784.4	Other speech disturbance	707.8	Chronic ulcer of other specified sites
785.9	Arterial bruit/weak pulse; other symptoms involving cardiovascular system	785.4	Gangrene
		903.00–903.9	Injury to blood vessels of upper ext.
900.0–900.9	Injury to blood vessels of head and neck	903.1	Injury to brachial blood vessel
900.01	Injury to common carotid artery	903.2	Injury to radial blood vessel
		903.3	Injury to ulnar blood vessel
900.02	Injury to external carotid artery	903.4	Injury to palmar artery
		904.0–904.9	Injury to blood vessels of lower ext./unspec.
900.03	Injury to internal carotid artery	904.0	Injury to common femoral artery
901.1	Injury to innominate & subclavian arteries	904.1	Injury to superficial femoral artery
996.1	Mechanical complication of vascular device, implant, or graft	904.2	Injury to femoral veins
		904.3	Injury to saphenous veins
		996.1	Mechanical complication of other vascular device, implant, or graft
996.70–996.79	Other complication of prosthetic device, implant, or graft	996.70–996.79	Other complication of internal prosthetic device, implant, or graft
996.73	Complications due to renal dialysis device, implant, or graft	996.73	Complication due to renal dialysis device, implant, or graft
998.0–998.9	Other complications of procedures not classified elsewhere		
998.11	Hemorrhage, hematoma, seroma complicating a procedure	998.1	Hemorrhage or hematoma complicating a procedure
		998.11	Hemorrhage, hematoma, seroma complicating a procedure
998.1	Accidental puncture during procedure		

Carotid duplex [CPT 93880, 92882]		*Arterial duplex [lower extremity 93925 (bilateral) and 93926 (unilateral), upper extremity 93930 (bilateral) and 93931 (unilateral)] and PVR [at rest only 93923, with exercise 93924, ABI 939221]*	
ICD-9	*Description*	*ICD-9*	*Description*
V58.49	Other specified aftercare following surgery	998.2	Accidental puncture or laceration during a procedure
		V58.49	Other specified aftercare following surgery

*Occlusion and stenosis require a fifth digit: 0, without infarction; 1, with infarction.

AA = aortic aneurysm; CVA = cerebrovascular accident; PVR = pulse volume recording; TIA = transient ischemic attack.

ICD-9 codes may change and, as such, these codes should be confirmed with the latest available coding update before being used for clinical purposes.

Venous duplex [CPT 93970 (bilateral) and 93971 (unilateral)]	
ICD-9	*Description*
415.11–415.19	Pulmonary embolism and infarction
451.0–451.9	Phlebitis and thrombophlebitis
451.0	Phlebitis and thrombophlebitis: superficial lower extremity
451.11	Phlebitis and thrombophlebitis: femoral
451.19	Phlebitis and thrombophlebitis: popliteal
451.81	Phlebitis and thrombophlebitis: iliac
451.82	Phlebitis and thrombophlebitis: superficial upper extremity
451.83	Phlebitis and thrombophlebitis: deep veins upper extremity
454.0	Varicose veins of lower extremities with ulcer
454.2	Varicose veins of lower extremities with inflammation and ulcer
459.1	Postphlebitic syndrome
459.2	Compression of vein
671.20–671.24	Superficial thrombophlebitis in pregnancy and puerperium
671.30–671.33	Deep thrombophlebitis, antepartum
671.40–671.44	Deep thrombophlebitis, postpartum
695.9	Unspecified erythematous condition
707.1	Ulcer of lower limbs except decubitus
729.5	Pain in limb
729.81	Swelling of limb
747.60–747.69	Other anomalies of peripheral vascular system
782.2	Localized superficial swelling, mass, or lump
782.3	Edema
785.4	Gangrene
786.0	Respiratory abnormality, unspecified
786.03	Apnea
786.04	Cheyne–Stokes respiration
786.05	Shortness of breath
786.06	Tachypnea
786.07	Wheezing
786.09	Other respiratory abnormality
786.3	Hemoptysis

Venous duplex [CPT 93970 (bilateral) and 93971 (unilateral)]	
ICD-9	*Description*
786.52	Painful respiration
786.59	Other discomfort, pressure, or tightness in chest
794.2	Nonspecific abnormal results of pulmonary function study
903.00–903.9	Injury to blood vessels of upper extremity
903.1	Injury to brachial blood vessel
903.2	Injury to radial blood vessel
903.3	Injury to ulnar blood vessel
903.4	Injury to palmar artery
904.0–904.9	Injury to vessels of lower extremity and unspecified sites
904.0	Injury to common femoral artery
904.1	Injury to superficial femoral artery
904.2	Injury to femoral veins
904.3	Injury to saphenous veins
996.1	Mechanical complication of other vascular device, implant, or graft
996.70–996.79	Other complications of internal prosthetic device, implant or graft
996.73	Complications due to renal dialysis device, implant, or graft
997.2	Peripheral vascular complications
998.2	Accidental puncture or laceration during a procedure
999.2	Other vascular complication of medical care
V45.81	Post-aortocoronary bypass status

ICD-9 codes may change and, as such, these codes should be confirmed with the latest available coding update before being used for clinical purposes.

Appendix 2: Example of Venous Duplex Protocol

Midwest Heart Specialists Vascular Laboratory lower extremity venous duplex protocol

Lower extremity venous duplex evaluation with color duplex imaging
Revised/approved date: 05/10/2004.

1 Purpose
To rule out or identify thrombosis in the veins of the lower extremities, and to identify the location and extent of the thrombus whenever possible. Duplex evaluation may also be used for the analysis of venous reflux and venous insufficiency.

2 Indications
2.1 Venous obstruction (symptomatic).
2.2 Leg pain of unknown etiology.
2.3 Swelling.
2.4 Possible pulmonary embolism.
2.5 Dyspnea.
2.6 Venous obstruction (asymptomatic).
2.7 Chronic leg ulcers or stasis.

3 Contraindications and limitations
3.1 Site trauma, such as open wounds over scan area.
3.2 Casts that cannot be removed or traction that limits access to the scan area.
3.3 Severe obesity.
3.4 Severe leg edema.
3.5 Patients who cannot be adequately positioned.

4 Equipment and supplies
4.1 High-resolution, real-time duplex unit and integrated, pulsed, range-gated Doppler, with or without color flow imaging. A 5–10 MHz transducer that allows visualization to 5–6 cm. Doppler color flow imaging is very helpful.
4.2 Continuous wave Doppler capability is optional.

4.3 Tilt table or bed that can produce a reversed Trendelenburg position.

4.4 Gel and optional gel warmer.

4.5 Face towels or paper hand towels for gel removal.

4.6 Material for hard copy documentation, e.g. videotape, color video printer, multi-image film, or digital archiving.

5 Patient preparation

5.1 Explain the procedure to the patient.

5.2 Have the patient disrobe from the waist down and put on a gown.

5.3 Place the patient on the table or bed in the supine position with the hip externally rotated and the knee slightly bent.

5.4 Document symptomatology or appropriate indications and other relevant medical history.

5.5 Place the bed or table in a reversed Trendelenburg position (head elevated about 20–30°) with the feet parallel. This is essential for proper examination of the patient to exclude or document thrombus.

5.6 To assess venous reflux and insufficiency, the patient should be in the standing position with adequate support available to ensure safety while scanning. Alternatively, the patient can be placed on a safe tilted examination table in a reversed Trendelenburg position at an angle of at least 30°. Appropriate safety measures, including a safe foot support, should be used to prevent the patient from sliding or falling.

5.7 The room should be warm. If the room is cool and the temperature cannot be regulated, warm the patient using heated blankets or other measures.

6 Procedure: general considerations

6.1 Proper vessel visualization. The vessel must be visualized clearly in a transverse view. It should appear round. (If not, check to ensure proper elevation of the bed or have the patient dangle his or her leg off the side of the bed.) The size of the vessels can also be affected by the position of the bed or the room temperature.

6.2 Full compression of the vein. Once the vein is visualized in a transverse view, light probe pressure is exerted directly over the vessel. If the vein contains no thrombus, it will collapse completely. If thrombus is present, echogenic material will usually be visualized within the lumen, and the thrombus will limit the compressibility of the vessel. If the vein is incompressible, but no echogenic material is visualized, more pressure is exerted over the vein. If the accompanying artery compresses and the vein does not, thrombus can be said to be present.

6.3 Doppler and color flow information. Optimal Doppler signals must be obtained, i.e. velocity, wall filter, and color must be set appropriately.

7 Procedure: test protocol

7.1 For outpatients, bilateral studies are performed for symptomatic patients, as it is well known that thrombotic disease does occur in asymptomatic limbs in patients with contralateral symptoms and/or risk factors.

7.2 For selected outpatients, if requested, a unilateral study may be performed under the following circumstances.

7.2.1 The patient is under 60 years of age and has no history of the following risk factors:

malignancy (other than nonmelanoma skin cancer);

pregnancy or within the first 6 weeks postpartum;

congestive heart failure;

symptomatic pulmonary disease;

morbid obesity;

cerebrovascular accident or other neurologic condition which limits ambulation significantly.

7.2.2 The patient has not had general anesthesia or abdominal, gynecologic, urologic, orthopedic, or neurologic surgery in the past 3 months.

7.2.3 The patient does not have a history of a prior deep vein thrombosis or pulmonary embolism.

7.2.4 The patient does not have a history of a known hematologic or serologic marker for increased thromboembolic disease, such as Factor V Leiden mutation, protein C deficiency, antithrombin III deficiency, lupus anticoagulant, anticardiolipin antibodies.

7.3 The venous study should not be unilateral if the patient's indication for the study is suspected pulmonary embolism.

7.4 If a unilateral study is performed under the above guidelines, insonation of the proximal contralateral femoral vein, demonstrating normal transverse compressions, AND assessment of venous respirophasicity with augmentation maneuvers should be carried out in all instances unless a contraindication exists. If this limited contralateral study is not normal, a full bilateral study should be performed.

8 Procedure: imaging protocol

8.1 Image the veins of the thigh. In the transverse plane, begin imaging at the inguinal ligament. This view is used in order to provide visualization of more than one vessel at a time and permits the most accurate assessment of vein wall compressibility. At this level, the confluence of the greater saphenous vein and the common femoral vein is visualized. The vein is differentiated from the artery by exerting light probe pressure. If it is thrombus free, the vein will compress by showing coapting of the sides of the vein with compression, while the artery will not. Use spectral Doppler and color flow imaging to assist in identifying the veins. Once the vessels have been properly identified, focus attention on compressing the vein to identify or rule out thrombus. If the vein compresses completely, it is thrombus free at that location (see Interpretation below). Compressions in the transverse view should be continued down the medial aspect of the thigh to the adductor canal, approximating the course of the femoral vein and the deep femoral vein (as much as is visible). Compressions should be approximately 1 cm apart. At this point, return to the groin and locate the saphenofemoral junction.

8.2   Image the greater saphenous vein. Follow the saphenous vein in transverse, compressing and releasing as you go, down the medial portion of the thigh until it takes an anterior turn just below the knee. Follow it near the tibia as it courses down the calf. Continue to follow it to the foot level just anterior to the medial malleolus. Because this vein is so superficial, it can be compressed easily by the weight of the probe resting on the skin. To prevent this, apply additional gel so that the probe glides easily along the gel-coated skin.

8.3   In the sagittal plane, visualize the saphenofemoral junction. Views with color flow and Doppler are then recorded, starting with the common femoral vein. Place the Doppler cursor in the common femoral vein and demonstrate the following flow patterns.

    8.3.1   Spontaneous flow that is detected without augmentation.

    8.3.2   Phasicity—waxing and waning of audible flow and spectral velocity in response to respiration.

    8.3.3   Competency—flow stops in response to a Valsalva maneuver or proximal and distal manual compression.

    8.3.4   Augmentation of the signal should be detected with distal limb compression, observing for signs of reversed flow that may be prolonged. If present, such a reflux signal should be measured with time calipers.

8.4   Record these color images and flow patterns in the superficial femoral vein and the greater saphenous vein, at the junction.

8.5   Image the popliteal vein. Place the transducer, in the transverse view, in the popliteal fossa and visualize the popliteal vein. Showing good compressibility, the vein is followed from the distal superficial femoral vein into the trifurcation.

8.6   Record the color images and flow patterns as described in 8.3 for the popliteal vein.

8.7   Image the veins of the calf.

    8.7.1   If the patient is able, help the patient to a sitting position with the legs dangling off the side of the bed. If the patient is unable to sit up, the legs can be externally rotated and the knees bent at an angle of 30°.

    8.7.2   Use the space between the Achilles tendon and the medial malleolus as a landmark to locate the posterior tibial veins. At this level, the veins are paired and accompanied by the posterior tibial artery. Perform transverse compression of these veins moving cephalad until reaching the tibial–peroneal trunk.

    8.7.3   A few inches up the posterior calf, the peroneal veins and artery are visible. They are located by identifying the fibula (a bright reflector about 3–5 cm deep in the calf). The peroneal veins are imaged just superficial to the fibula from a medial projection. Compression of these veins is performed while moving toward the tibial–peroneal trunk.

    8.7.4   Demonstrate flow in the posterior tibial veins using color flow and Doppler. Record phasicity, distal augmentation, and competence.

    8.7.5   Place the transducer in the popliteal fossa to examine the deep muscle calf veins (medial and lateral gastrocnemius veins, and soleal sinusoids). Compression in a transverse view should be documented.

8.7.6 The lesser saphenous vein joins the popliteal vein most commonly at the popliteal fossa. Follow the lesser saphenous vein distally to the posterior surface of the calf, if possible, until it passes between the lateral malleolus and the Achilles tendon. Document and record compression and flow information using color imaging and Doppler.

Note. Signals at the posterior tibial veins (and other calf veins) may not be spontaneous or phasic.

8.8 For the analysis of varicosities and the assessment of venous insufficiency, the patient's deep and superficial venous system should be examined in the standing position. This examination should include the following.

8.8.1 Common femoral vein just proximal to the saphenofemoral junction.

8.8.2 Femoral vein at mid-thigh (superficial femoral vein).

8.8.3 Popliteal vein.

8.8.4 Greater saphenous vein at the saphenofemoral junction; two additional locations between the saphenofemoral junction and the mid-thigh, and another sample below the knee.

8.8.5 Lesser saphenous vein at its junction with the popliteal vein or distal femoral vein and in the mid-portion of the posterior calf.

8.8.6 A search for prominent perforating veins medially in the leg, connecting the superficial veins to the deep system. They are located in the distal thigh, just below the knee, and in the Cockett's region at the level of the ankle.

9 Documentation

9.1 The examination is performed with the videotape running to ensure that the entire examination is documented. The name of the patient is entered on the screen, as are the date of the examination and the examination being performed. Each videotape is numbered for easy reference.

9.2 Color photographs are taken of selected points of interest in order to augment the videotape documentation of the examination and to provide summary information for referring physicians, as well as a quick reference for the reading physician. Vessel identification and the pathology identified are annotated on these photographs.

9.3 A brief history sheet is filled out for each examination, including the name of the patient, patient number, the date of the examination, the referring physician, and other information deemed pertinent.

9.4. A venous duplex worksheet is completed that indicates that signals were heard in the common femoral, superficial femoral, popliteal, and posterior tibial veins. In the presence of thrombus, the extent and location are indicated on this worksheet. All other pathology is likewise indicated on this sheet.

9.5 Any technical difficulties encountered during the examination that may influence its diagnostic quality should also be noted.

9.6 The technologist must sign or initial the worksheet to indicate which technologist performed the examination.

9.7 When needed, a preliminary report sheet is completed for each patient. The impression given to the referring physician is summarized here. The physician receiving the report, the impression given, and the technologist making the report are recorded on this form.

9.8 The aforementioned sheets are compiled into the patient chart, which is kept on file for a minimum of 3 years.

10   Interpretation

10.1 Normal Doppler signals.

10.1.1 Spontaneous and phasic signals are heard at all levels except at the calf, where signals may or may not be spontaneous or phasic.

10.1.2 Distal compression of the limb augments the Doppler signals.

10.2 Abnormal Doppler signals.

10.2.1 When venous Doppler signals are absent, obstruction of the vein at that level is suspected.

10.2.2 When a signal is present, but is continuous, proximal obstruction or extrinsic compression is suspected.

10.2.3 When distal compression does not augment the venous signal, obstruction distal to the probe and proximal to the compression is suspected.

10.2.4 Weak or dampened augmentation suggests total or partial obstruction of the veins distal to the probe and proximal to the compression.

10.2.5 Reflux may be said to be present when the refluxing signal is **greater than** the following:

0.5 s in the greater saphenous vein or lesser saphenous vein;

0.5 s in the femoral or popliteal veins;

0.4 s in the perforators.

Note: Normal Doppler signals may be present when thrombus is non-obstructive.

10.3 Normal imaging observations.

10.3.1 When imaging the vein in a transverse plane, the vein is first observed for the presence or absence of visible echogenic material. If none is visualized, the vein is compressed using probe pressure. If the vein collapses completely and no echogenic material is visualized, the vein is thrombus free at that location. Color will fill the vein completely in response to distal limb compression.

10.4 Abnormal imaging observations.

10.4.1 Thrombus is said to be present when echogenic material is visualized within the vein, and compression of the vein is observed to be limited by the contained thrombus.

10.4.2 The color moves around the echogenic material with distal limb compression if the thrombus is not fully occlusive.

10.4.3 The vein is occluded: no flow is identified within the vessel.

Note: In some views, color flow may appear to cover a nonobstructive thrombus, especially if color gains are set too high.

10.4.4 If no echogenic material is visualized, but the vein does not fully compress with light probe pressure, more pressure is exerted. If the adjacent artery compresses and the vein does not, thrombus is likely to be present. Color flow imaging can be used to confirm this.

10.4.5 Once thrombus is identified, attention is focused on the characteristics of the thrombus.

Acute thrombus:

- is most often lightly echogenic or hypoechoic;
- may be poorly attached to the vein wall;
- often dilates the vein wall (if the vein is totally acutely obstructed).

Chronic thrombus (defined as thrombus likely to be older than 6 weeks of age) most often will:

- appear more brightly echogenic;
- be attached to the vein wall;
- be associated with a not so dilated vein diameter;
- contract the vein wall over time (if totally obstructed);
- often be accompanied by collateral veins nearby; color Doppler is especially useful in visualizing such collaterals;
- not have a "tip" which is seen to move to-and-fro with respiration;
- likely to have some recanalization, as evidenced by variably prominent interspersed color Doppler signals laced between echogeneity of the remaining thrombus material.

11 Reporting

11.1 When an examination of an outpatient has been completed, the preliminary impression is telephoned or faxed to the referring physician while the patient is getting dressed. Ideally, the technologist speaks directly with the physician before the patient is allowed to leave. If the results show no evidence of thrombus and the physician is not available, the patient may leave and await subsequent instructions from the ordering or treating physician. If the physician is not available and the results are positive for deep vein thrombosis, the technologist must either find a way to contact the physician or contact another physician regarding appropriate treatment. The medical director should become involved as necessary to help ensure proper care of the patient.

11.2 If the venous study is performed on an inpatient, the physician is called in a timely fashion, and a note is placed in the chart.

11.3 The study is reviewed by the medical director or reading physician, and an official report is dictated. The dictation is transcribed, and the report is returned to the medical director or reading physician for his/her signature, or an electronic signature.

11.4 A copy of the signed report is sent to the referring physician and/or a copy is placed in the chart.

11.5 A copy of the final report is placed in the patient's laboratory chart together with the technical worksheets. The chart is filed in medical records.

12 Cleaning and care of equipment

12.1 The transducers are wiped clean of gel and disinfected after each use.

12.2 Whenever blood, body fluids, or possibly infected materials come into contact with the probe, it is cleaned as directed by the manufacturer following universal precautions and safety protocols.

12.3 Clean linen is placed on the examination table after each patient examination. Soiled linen is disposed of properly.

Index

Page numbers in *italics* refer to figures and those in **bold** to tables; please note that figures and tables are only indicated when they are separated from their text references. Index entries are filed in letter-by-letter alphabetical order.